SpringerBriefs in Public Health

Child Health

Series Editor
Angelo P. Giardino, Houston, TX, USA

SpringerBriefs in Public Health present concise summaries of cutting-edge research and practical applications from across the entire field of public health, with contributions from medicine, bioethics, health economics, public policy, biostatistics, and sociology.

The focus of the series is to highlight current topics in public health of interest to a global audience, including health care policy; social determinants of health; health issues in developing countries; new research methods; chronic and infectious disease epidemics; and innovative health interventions.

Featuring compact volumes of 50 to 125 pages, the series covers a range of content from professional to academic. Possible volumes in the series may consist of timely reports of state-of-the art analytical techniques, reports from the field, snapshots of hot and/or emerging topics, elaborated theses, literature reviews, and in-depth case studies. Both solicited and unsolicited manuscripts are considered for publication in this series.

Briefs are published as part of Springer's eBook collection, with millions of users worldwide. In addition, Briefs are available for individual print and electronic purchase.

Briefs are characterized by fast, global electronic dissemination, standard publishing contracts, easy-to-use manuscript preparation and formatting guidelines, and expedited production schedules. We aim for publication 8-12 weeks after acceptance.

More information about this series at http://www.springer.com/series/10138

Hans B. Kersten • Andrew F. Beck
Melissa Klein

Editors

Identifying and Addressing Childhood Food Insecurity in Healthcare and Community Settings

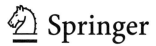 Springer

Editors
Hans B. Kersten
St. Christopher's Hospital for Children
Drexel University College of Medicine
Philadelphia, PA, USA

Melissa Klein
Cincinnati Children's Hospital Medical
Center
University of Cincinnati College of
Medicine
Cincinnati, OH, USA

Andrew F. Beck
Cincinnati Children's Hospital Medical
Center
University of Cincinnati College of
Medicine
Cincinnati, OH, USA

SpringerBriefs in Child Health

ISSN 2192-3698   ISSN 2192-3701   (electronic)
SpringerBriefs in Public Health
ISBN 978-3-319-76047-6   ISBN 978-3-319-76048-3   (eBook)
https://doi.org/10.1007/978-3-319-76048-3

Library of Congress Control Number: 2018938173

Printed on acid-free paper

This Springer imprint is published by the registered company Springer International Publishing AG part of Springer Nature.
The registered company address is: Gewerbestrasse 11, 6330 Cham, Switzerland

Contents

Contributors

Andrew F. Beck Cincinnati Children's Hospital Medical Center and University of Cincinnati College of Medicine, Cincinnati, OH, USA

Janine S. Bruce Stanford University School of Medicine, Stanford, CA, USA

Kelly A. Courts St. Christopher's Hospital for Children, Drexel University, Philadelphia, PA, USA

Kofi Essel Children's National Health System, The George Washington University School of Medicine & Health Sciences, Washington, DC, USA

Baraka D. Floyd Stanford School of Medicine, Stanford, CA, USA

Adrienne W. Henize Cincinnati Children's Hospital Medical Center and University of Cincinnati College of Medicine, Cincinnati, OH, USA

Hans B. Kersten St. Christopher's Hospital for Children, Drexel University College of Medicine, Philadelphia, PA, USA

Melissa Klein Cincinnati Children's Hospital Medical Center and University of Cincinnati College of Medicine, Cincinnati, OH, USA

Deepak Palakshappa Wake Forest School of Medicine, Winston-Salem, NC, USA

Chapter 1
Epidemiology and Pathophysiology of Food Insecurity

Kofi Essel and Kelly A. Courts

Abbreviations

ASEC	Annual Social and Economic Supplement (report)
CPS	Current Population Survey
DHHS	Department of Health and Human Services
FI	Food Insecurity
FPL	Federal Poverty Level
HFSSM	Household Food Security Survey Module
LSRO	Life Sciences Research Office
NHANES	National Health and Nutrition Examination Survey
NNMRR	National Nutrition Monitoring and Related Research Act
SDH	Social Determinants of Health
USDA	United States Department of Agriculture

Aims
1. Define key terms, including FI, hunger, and the SDH.
2. Outline the history of FI measurement in the U.S.
3. Describe the key tools that are currently used to measure FI in the U.S.
4. Discuss the trends and current epidemiology of FI in the U.S.
5. Discuss the pathophysiology of FI and its links to health outcomes originating in childhood.

K. Essel (✉)
Children's National Health System, The George Washington University School of Medicine & Health Sciences, Washington, DC, USA
e-mail: kessel@childrensnational.org

K. A. Courts
St. Christopher's Hospital for Children, Drexel University, Philadelphia, PA, USA

© The Author(s) 2018
H. B. Kersten et al. (eds.), *Identifying and Addressing Childhood Food Insecurity in Healthcare and Community Settings*, SpringerBriefs in Public Health, https://doi.org/10.1007/978-3-319-76048-3_1

Food Insecurity as a Social Determinant of Health

At the core of western society lies a deeply held belief that children should not suffer, that they be given all opportunities to thrive and develop in a supportive and enriching environment. In reality, many children do not have such opportunities, and there exists inherent inequities that may affect a child's health and well-being from their early years extending across the life-course. Current medical practice strives to prevent acute disease and buffer the progression of chronic disease. Increasingly, these objectives are pushing physicians and other clinicians and medical professionals toward acknowledgement of the complete array of risk factors that children might experience, including those factors or stressors that can become "toxic."

"Toxic stress" results from persistent exposures that incite physiologic hormonal responses. When these stressors do not diminish, and without co-existent adequate buffers, the stress response cannot be effectively shut down [1]. This can result in less effective neurologic and immunologic responses, prompting cognitive impairment, acute illnesses, and morbidity resulting from chronic disease processes [1, 2]. Social, economic, and environmental factors frequently underlie these stressors. As a result, the conditions in which individuals live, work, play, grow, and age, the so-called social determinants of health (SDH), are increasingly recognized as vital to health and well-being [3]. These SDH influence the severity and consistency of stress exposures, driving health outcomes that include premature death. Given disparities in how these stressors, and the SDH in general, are experienced across populations, disparities in those outcomes result [4]. With growing evidence highlighting the linkages between the SDH and "toxic" outcomes, clinicians are increasingly turning toward socially-minded, community-connected approaches to care provision. Indeed, clinicians must be able to address more than just the clinical disease state of a patient; they, too, must acknowledge and then address those upstream factors that influence the health of their patients.

One such factor is food insecurity (FI), defined as "the limited or uncertain availability of nutritionally adequate and safe foods or limited or uncertain ability to acquire acceptable foods in socially acceptable ways" [5]. FI is a distinctly different phenomenon than hunger. FI is typically examined at the household level, while hunger is an individual's sensation of pain or discomfort associated with food deprivation [6]. Hunger may result from FI but is not necessarily the most persistent or severe result of being food insecure. Although hunger is a recognizable and accepted term used by many advocates, we will aim to provide a more technical description and distinguish these terms for the reader [7].

Historical Context of FI

Before the late 1960s, barring the Great Depression years, hunger and FI were not widely viewed as significant public health issues in the U.S. Consensus was lacking on both definition and measurement making the true extent of the issue hard to determine and quantify. The airing of the CBS documentary, "Hunger in America," following a visit by the Senate Subcommittee on Employment, Manpower and Poverty to the Mississippi Delta, brought the issue more directly into the public discourse. Not until the 1980s, however, when economic conditions and the media increased attention on the issue, did the question of whether hunger widely existed in the U.S. come to the fore with then-President Reagan initiating a "Task Force on Food Assistance" to investigate the prevalence of hunger and the effectiveness of national food assistance programs. Their 1984 report indicated that hunger, defined as individuals experiencing personalized undernutrition, was not widespread in the U.S.; however, hunger, defined as a social phenomenon in which individuals may have an "inability, even occasionally" to access adequate food, was present. In addition, the report stressed the need for a more direct, objective measurement of hunger, as opposed to the indirect measures like poverty and unemployment that had traditionally been used [8].

As a result, researchers and advocates began to develop and test survey measures to more accurately identify the problem. In 1990, a seminal report influenced by an ad hoc expert panel and completed by the Life Sciences Research Office (LSRO) of the Federation of American Societies for Experimental Biology created the consensus conceptual definitions for "FI" and "hunger" while also developing a consistent platform for future research [5, 8, 9]. In 1992, following the passage of the National Nutrition Monitoring and Related Research Act (NNMRR), the USDA and Department of Health and Human Services (DHHS) brought together representatives from federal agencies, academic researchers, and members of private organizations, among others, to form the Federal Food Security Measurement Project. This group reached agreement on key issues related to the best approach for national measurement of FI. Finally, in 1995, after field testing and revisions, standardized measures of FI were incorporated into the Census Bureau's "Current Population Survey" (CPS) as the "Food Security Supplement" (FSS) [8].

Measurement of FI

The USDA has subsequently been able to report the nation's annual food security statistics since 1995. Sponsored and funded by the USDA's Economic Research Service (ERS) and conducted by the U.S. Census Bureau, this is considered the gold standard summary report [6]. The CPS collects monthly data on approximately 50,000 households chosen to be representative of state and national civilian, noninstitutionalized populations within the U.S [6, 8, 10]. The FSS (within the CPS) measures: (1) the nation's food security statistics with the Household Food Security Survey Module (HFSSM); (2) household food expenditures; and (3) use of food and nutritional assistance programs by FI households [6, 8].

The HFSSM, composed of 18 total questions, is designed to provide a precise measure of the nation's food security status (Table 1.1). The first 3 questions relate to the household in general. The next 7 are designed to determine the FI status of

Table 1.1 U.S. Household Food Security Survey Module: 18-item questionnaire used to assess food security status of households [6]

Questions related to the household in general	1. "We worried whether our food would run out before we got money to buy more." Was that often, sometimes, or never true for you in the last 12 months?
	2. "The food that we bought just didn't last and we didn't have money to get more." Was that often, sometimes, or never true for you in the last 12 months?
	3. "We couldn't afford to eat balanced meals." Was that often, sometimes, or never true for you in the last 12 months?
Questions designed to determine food insecurity status of adults living within the household	4. In the last 12 months, did you or other adults in the household ever cut the size of your meals or skip meals because there wasn't enough money for food? (Yes/No)
	5. (If yes to question 4) How often did this happen—almost every month, some months but not every month, or in only 1 or 2 months?
	6. In the last 12 months, did you ever eat less than you felt you should because there wasn't enough money for food? (Yes/No)
	7. In the last 12 months, were you ever hungry, but didn't eat because there wasn't enough money for food? (Yes/No)
	8. In the last 12 months, did you lose weight because there wasn't enough money for food? (Yes/No)
	9. In the last 12 months did you or other adults in your household ever not eat for a whole day because there wasn't enough money for food? (Yes/No)
	10. (If yes to question 9) How often did this happen—almost every month, some months but not every month, or in only 1 or 2 months? (Questions 11–18 were asked only if the household included children age 0–17)
Questions designed to determine food insecurity status of children living within the household	11. "We relied on only a few kinds of low-cost food to feed our children because we were running out of money to buy food." Was that often, sometimes, or never true for you in the last 12 months?
	12. "We couldn't feed our children a balanced meal, because we couldn't afford that." Was that often, sometimes, or never true for you in the last 12 months?
	13. "The children were not eating enough because we just couldn't afford enough food." Was that often, sometimes, or never true for you in the last 12 months?
	14. In the last 12 months, did you ever cut the size of any of the children's meals because there wasn't enough money for food? (Yes/No)
	15. In the last 12 months, were the children ever hungry but you just couldn't afford more food? (Yes/No)
	16. In the last 12 months, did any of the children ever skip a meal because there wasn't enough money for food? (Yes/No)
	17. (If yes to question 16) How often did this happen—almost every month, some months but not every month, or in only 1 or 2 months?
	18. In the last 12 months, did any of the children ever not eat for a whole day because there wasn't enough money for food? (Yes/No)

those adults that are living within the household. The final 8 questions are asked only if a child is present in the household, assessing food security status of those children from the parent's perspective. Each question refers to the past 12 months and indicates a lack of money as the reason for the behavior or concern in order to ensure that the food shortage is not related to voluntary fasting or dieting [6, 10]. Any household with an income at or below 185% of the federal poverty level (FPL) is asked these HFSSM questions. Those above 185% of the FPL are asked only if they respond positively on either of two preliminary food access questions [6].

Questions within the HFSSM are designed to gradually progress in severity along four discrete phases of a household's lived experience (Fig. 1.1). These phases involve: (1) "Food Anxiety" in which individuals have an increased worry, anxiety or preoccupation with food availability; (2) "Monotony of Diet" in which the household diet declines in quality, desirability, and variety; (3) "Adult Restriction" in which adults experience an inadequate food supply and try to protect children at all costs; and (4) "Child Restriction" in which children experience an inadequate food supply and household members may attempt to gather food in what some describe as more "socially unacceptable" ways (i.e., utilization of food pantries or emergency kitchens, through bartering or illegal activity) [8, 9, 11–14]. The HFSSM tool therefore focuses on the uncertainty and insufficiency of food availability and access along with household behaviors or responses to FI. That said, the tool intentionally does not measure other aspects of FI such as nutritional adequacy, quality of diet, safety of foods, or management/coping strategies (acceptable, unacceptable, legal, illegal) to counteract FI [8, 10, 15]. It should be noted that the HFSSM, and the FSS more generally, collects data from 1 adult respondent per household in noninstitutionalized populations. It does, therefore, omit certain vulnerable populations that may experience FI, such as the homeless and residents of institutionalized settings (e.g., jails, group homes, and hospitals) [6].

Households that answer with more than 2 positive/affirmative responses on the HFSSM are considered "food insecure"(Table 1.2). Households that respond with 0 positive/affirmative responses are considered to have "high food security." There is also a special category labeled as "marginally food secure," inclusive of those households with 1 or 2 positive/affirmative responses. Marginally food secure households may resemble households that are either food secure or insecure, but studies have still shown significant associations between marginal status and adverse health outcomes, including for children [16, 17]. Households can

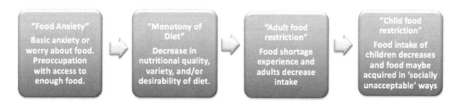

Fig. 1.1 Example of the spectrum of food insecurity that can affect a household or family

Table 1.2 USDA definitions and prevalence of food security for households with children in 2016

USDA designation	Number of affirmative responses to HFSSM questions	USDA definition	2016 prevalence
Household food security status for households with children			
High food security	0 of 18	No reported indications of food-access problems or limitations.	73.28%
Marginal food security	1–2 of 18	Few reported indications—typically of anxiety over food sufficiency or shortage of food in the house. Little or no indication of changes in diets or food intake.	10.21%
			Total Household Food Security: 83.49%
			32.1 million households w/ children
			~60.9 million US children
Low food security	3–7 of 18	Reports of reduced quality, variety, or desirability of diet. Little or no indication of reduced food intake.	11.72%
Very low food security	8 or more of 18	Reports of multiple indications of disrupted eating patterns, such as skipping meals, and reduced food intake.	4.79%
			Total Household Food Insecurity: 16.51%
			6.34 million households w/ children
			~12.9 million US children
Child food security status for households with children			
Food insecurity among Children	2 or more of 8 child centered questions	Caregivers report that one or more child in the household lacked adequate, nutritious food at times during the year.	7.21%
Very low food security among children	5 or more of 8 child centered questions	Caregivers reported that children were hungry, skipped a meal, or did not eat for a whole day because there was not enough money for food.	0.78%
			Total Child Food Insecurity: 7.99%
			~3.1 million US children

Source: USDA, Economic Research Service, data from the 2016 Current Population Survey Food Security Supplement [6, 17]

also be broken down into low food security and very low food security based on the number of positive/affirmative responses. Low food security refers to those households that experience food access concerns and reduced diet quality, but with very little to no episodes of decreased food intake. Households with very low food security have documented episodes of decreased food intake and disrupted eating patterns (See Chap. 4 for further discussion of how these definitions materialize in real-life situations) [6].

Alternative Measures of FI

The placement of both the FSS and the HFSSM tools in the U.S. Census Bureau's CPS provide reliable and validated means through which FI can be nationally estimated and tracked over time [8, 18]. The HFSSM tool and its variations have also been incorporated into other federal government surveys as part of the Federal Food Security Measurement Project in order to establish a more robust measure of the degree of FI across the country [8].

Other national surveys use the USDA data or similar collection strategies to gain a better sense of FI rates in the U.S. Feeding America's Map the Meal Gap Report is one such example. Feeding America is a non-profit organization that serves as the largest hunger-relief agency in the U.S [19]. Their annual survey, launched in 2011, uses FSS and HFSSM national and state data, along with other data sets (e.g., the U.S. Census' American Community Survey and data from the Bureau of Labor Statistics). Through this data, Feeding America is able to quantify FI rates down to the county level [19, 20]. Such information, available from the federal and non-profit sources, allows advocacy groups, state and local governments, and local communities to be more strategic in how resources are provided to often-hidden, food insecure populations.

National Trends in FI Rates

Initially, between 1995 and 2000, the FSS survey was collected during different seasons so as to allow researchers to understand seasonal variation in FI patterns [8]. This led to the determination that summer months (July–September) experienced a greater prevalence of FI than March–April and November–December [21–23]. In 2001, the USDA changed their approach, opting to conduct their surveys in December of each year. This allowed for more consistent measurement of trends from year to year, while limiting the effect of seasonal variation.

The latest USDA Household Food Security report, conducted in 2016, indicated that 12.3% of households (15.5 million total households with an estimated 41.2 million people) were food insecure at some point during the preceding year. Figure 1.2 shows national FI trends since 2001. During the Great Recession of 2007–2009, the

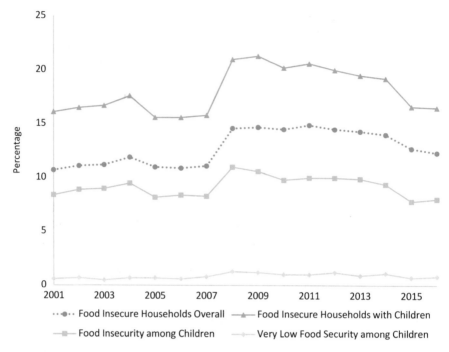

Fig. 1.2 Trends in prevalence of food insecurity in U.S. households between 2001 and 2016. (Source: USDA, Economic Research Service, data from the 2016 Current Population Survey Food Security Supplement [6])

prevalence of FI spiked, reaching its highest rates between 2008 and 2011. After peaking in 2011, when 14.9% of households were classified as FI, there began a gradual downward trend. Still, the current prevalence of 12.3% has not yet reached the 2007 pre-recession level of 11.1%. Households with children have continued to experience higher rates of FI than the overall population. The highest rates of childhood FI also occurred between 2008 and 2011, peaking in 2009 when 21.3% of households with children were classified as food insecure. There has been a gradual downward trend paralleling that of the general population, moving to its current rate of 16.5% (6.3 million households; estimated 12.9 million children) [6].

In the U.S., FI is more often described as episodic or cyclical than chronic. On average, although roughly 25% of food insecure households are thought to experience FI during every month of a year, generally, households that experienced FI at any time during 2016 were food insecure for an estimated 7 out of 12 months [6]. This episodic hardship may lead to what some experts describe as a "decreased cognitive bandwidth." In other words, a preoccupation with identifying when and where one's next meal will be may limit one's ability to focus on other cognitively consuming tasks such as health maintenance and chronic disease management [24, 25].

There is an episodic nature to FI prevalence within years and across years. Two longitudinal studies directed by the ERS looked at household-level FI rates over multiple years, finding that the majority of FI-classified households are only truly food insecure for 1 year out of many [26, 27]. While some households certainly do experience FI across years, it is more common for households to cycle in and out of FI over time (i.e., food insecure 1 year but not the next). As a result, an increased awareness of and focus on identifying newly food insecure households is critical for quickly addressing the problem, limiting its chronicity, and improving a family's bandwidth.

There are also questions regarding how severely children are affected by household FI regardless of whether it is persistent or cyclical. As raised earlier, children may be buffered from FI by their parents, or other adults within the household. Typically, just half of households with children classified as experiencing FI report that children within the household are directly affected (See Fig. 1.3). According to the USDA, approximately 8% of households with children have FI severe enough to result in food shortages that affect those children (3 million households; estimated 6.5 million children) [6]. Thus, many families cannot completely shield all children from their limited food supply. In addition, the actual burden of FI in children is

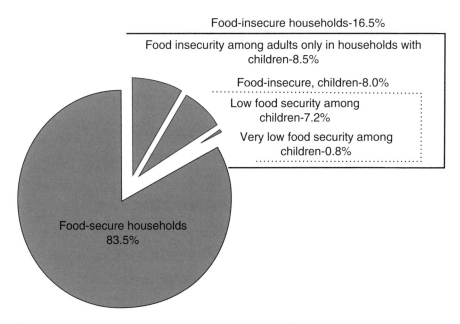

Fig. 1.3 U.S. food insecurity prevalence for U.S. households with children according to the USDA. (Adapted from USDA, Economic Research Service, data from the 2016 Current Population Survey Food Security Supplement. U.S. households with children by food security status of adults and children, 2016. [Image on Internet]. 2017 [updated 2017 Oct 4; cited 2017 December 1]. Available from: https://www.ers.usda.gov/topics/food-nutrition-assistance/food-security-in-the-us/key-statistics-graphics/ [6])

likely increased due to the inability of families to shield them from the psychosocial stressors associated with FI regardless of whether actual food shortages reach the child [28–32].

FI is a problem that typically burdens populations with income fragility, with few resources, or with a limited social network. Such populations have fewer supports to turn to in times of need, times where their ability to access or afford nutritious foods is diminished. A deeper understanding of these risk factors, developed below, is critical in the identification of strategies to confront such a pervasive problem.

Risk Factors for FI

The USDA identifies multiple risk factors for household FI (Fig. 1.4). In addition to households with children, risks also include single parent-headed households, households headed by racial/ethnic minorities, and low-income households. Evidence also suggests that those living in the Southern U.S., those in cities, and

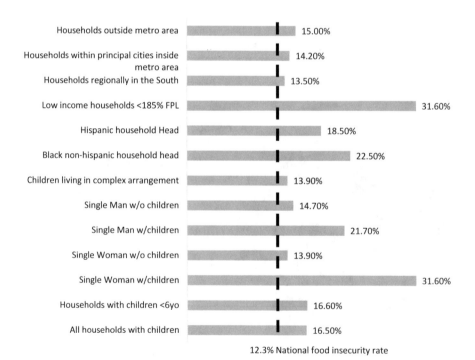

Fig. 1.4 Households with an average prevalence of food insecurity that is higher than the national average, 2016. (Source: USDA, Economic Research Service, data from the 2016 Current Population Survey Food Security Supplement [6])

those in more rural communities are also at heightened risk. According to the 2017 CPS Annual Social and Economic Supplement (ASEC) report, almost 40% (28.7 million) of children younger than 18 years lived in households described as "poor, near poor, or low income" (income below 200% of FPL). Nearly 18% (13.2 million) of children lived in households described as "poor" (income below 100% FPL) with another 8.2% (6 million) of children living in "deep" poverty (income below 50% FPL) [33]. These economic conditions, a preponderance of child poverty or near-poverty, likely underpins racial and ethnic disparities: 22% and 19.4% of African-Americans and Hispanics, respectively, live below the FPL compared to just 11% of Whites [33]. Given that such under-represented minorities experience the highest rates of poverty, it is not a surprise that they also experience excessively high rates of FI [6, 33].

Household income is among the biggest factors contributing to FI; it is inherent to the definition of FI and is embedded in many of the measurement tools. This confluence of FI and poverty is apparent in FSS data. National trends indicate that nearly 60% of all food insecure households and 65% of food insecure households with children, have an income less than 185% of the FPL. Households in poverty (income below 100% FPL) make up 34% of all food insecure households and 38% of food insecure households with children [6]. Children in low income households are especially vulnerable to FI even as parents adapt to limited food supplies. Indeed, some parents report the need for strategies to stretch their food supply, including watering down infant formulas, selling or bartering personal property, buying cheaper foods that may be less nutritious, buying poorly packaged foods such as dented or damaged packages, or eating food after expiration [34–37].

These practices can exist at other income levels as poverty alone does not always equate to living in a food insecure household. Indeed, households with incomes well above the FPL can also experience FI. Nearly 1 in 4 (24.3%) households, and 1 in 5 (19.2%) households with children, reported incomes >185% FPL while also experiencing FI in the preceding 12 months [6]. Factors such as changes in composition of the household, uneven income during the course of a year, unexpected or unusually high economic needs, or a lack of shared resources within a household have all been shown to contribute to FI, even for those with higher incomes [38].

There are other factors that can be protective. For example, households with a heightened degree of social capital (i.e., having family or friends to turn to in times of need), more wealth and liquid assets to fall back on, stable housing situations, stable health status of household members, and consistently accessible sources of affordable and nutritious foods may all fare better [9, 36, 37, 39]. Also, federal nutrition programs often serve as an anchor for families to buffer the threats of poverty (further discussed in Chap. 3). These programs can be critical for eligible households; those with higher incomes may not qualify [6]. Thus, many will come to rely on emergency kitchens and food pantries that may be inaccessible and insufficient for quality nutrition for the household [6, 17]. When protective factors are not in place, or when they are elusive, households and key sub-populations discussed below may find themselves at higher risk for continued experience with FI, being unable to buffer the socioeconomic challenges and negative economic shocks that acutely burden them.

Special Populations

Although 1 in 6 U.S. households with children experience FI, there are many subpopulations that warrant special attention considering their heightened risk for FI severity and depth [20, 40, 41]. We highlight three example subpopulations below: teenagers, college students, and immigrant families.

Teenagers

As discussed above, parents often attempt to shield children from challenges associated with FI [12, 42]. Generally, parents indicate that older children and teenagers are also shielded from FI's effects; however, studies that have asked these older children directly about food access and availability within their households suggest that parents frequently, perhaps unknowingly, underreport the challenges that extend to their children [32, 43]. These children, frequently teenagers, often indicate that they are aware of their household's FI and use their own coping strategies to decrease or alter their food intake to protect their younger siblings or parents. They often do this without their parent's knowledge [32, 44]. Some also report asking for less food at meal time, purposely not asking for certain types of food at a grocery store, attempting to stretch their meals, asking members of their social network for money or food, selling items to gain money, and engaging in criminal behavior, including sex trafficking [32, 45]. Although the data are mixed in the degree of misreporting from parents, this population is clearly at risk and may be more burdened by their household's FI than previously thought [46–50].

College Students

Many of these teenagers become college students, who themselves represent another at-risk population. There is emerging evidence linking FI on college campuses to potentially unhealthy coping strategies, poor health, and academic challenges [51–55]. College students can have a lack of consistent income or employment, low paying jobs, academic and social stressors, and, occasionally, housing instability [55]. Coping behaviors or strategies that may be unique to college students include relying on food or money from social networks, living with their parents instead of the dormitory, accessing food banks or pantries, acquiring high interest loans, or accruing debt on credit cards. Others may seek out higher paying jobs, potentially at the expense of their studies. These strategies, though potentially helpful in the short term, could increase the stress felt by the student, potentially worsening or deepening the cycle of FI in the longer term [56]. Not surprisingly, these experiences are then associated with negative health and academic outcomes, including a higher likelihood of anxiety and depression, and a lower grade-point average [52, 54, 57].

Immigrant Populations

Immigrants have a higher prevalence of FI compared to non-immigrants. This is thought to result from many factors, including increased financial constraints, decreased eligibility or ability to access federal nutrition programs, and cultural barriers [28, 58, 59]. A 2012 report from the University of Kentucky indicated that children in immigrant families are at higher risk for experiencing very low food security; such children make up 40% of all those that experience the deepest levels of FI [60]. Another study indicated that children living in households with foreign-born mothers were 3-times more likely than those with native-born mothers to experience very low food security after controlling for factors including marital status, educational attainment, and employment status [61]. Not surprisingly, these same children are also significantly more likely to experience fair or poor health (compared to good or very good health) [28]. Self-reported health outcomes are just one example of the many ways FI has been shown to effect health and well-being, a discussion that follows below.

FI and Health Outcomes

The associations between FI and child health have been abundantly researched and generally fall into three categories: physical, mental/psychosocial, and academic/developmental outcomes [41]. The sections that follow highlight key evidence for links to outcomes in each of these categories, supporting the importance of addressing FI in childhood to avoid a trajectory of negative outcomes along the life-course. It is important to remember that FI may more often be invisible and not consistently identified by clinical signs or symptoms [62].

Physical Health

Children living in food insecure households are generally in poorer health than their food secure peers [63]. They get sick more often, recover more slowly, and are hospitalized more frequently [64]. FI has been specifically associated with micronutrient deficiencies including anemia, morbidity resulting from chronic diseases like asthma, and poor oral health [65–68]. The relationship between obesity, which currently effects about 18.5% of our nation's children, and FI has proven complex and less definitive [69].

FI and obesity have both been shown to be directly associated with race and socioeconomic status [6, 69, 70]. In 1995, a case report was published by Dr. William Dietz that suggested the possibility of a paradoxical relationship between FI and unintended weight gain [71]. Many have referred to this potential relationship as an "obesity paradox." There have been multiple hypotheses advanced as theoretical underpinnings of such a counter-intuitive relationship. Indeed, some have suggested that weight increases could stem from overconsumption of nutrient-poor/energy-dense foods, cycles of overeating and food deprivation, decreased opportunities for physical activity, and increased stress levels and hormonal imbalance [72–76]. However, the evidence linking these two phenomena together in children continues to be mixed. Some studies indicate a positive association [29, 77–80], some a negative association [81–83], and some indicate no such association [84–86]. While continued research is necessary to more deeply understand the association between FI and obesity, the evidence linking them both to disadvantaged populations is clear and provides a target for effective joint interventions.

The literature on healthcare access and utilization for children in food insecure households is also mixed. Cross-sectional data has shown FI to be independently associated with having no usual primary care source, postponed medical care, postponed medications, and not receiving the recommended well-child care visits [87]. However, other studies were unable to replicate these findings and instead found no significant associations [88, 89].

Mental and Psychosocial Health

FI's association with negative mental health outcomes is supported by a body of evidence. Children in food insecure households have higher odds of experiencing adverse emotional symptoms, including feeling low, irritable, and nervous, while also reporting greater life dissatisfaction [90]. FI is strongly associated with both depression and suicidal ideation during childhood and later in life [91, 92], suggesting prevention of early FI may be of particular importance for mental health across the life-course [93].

Behavioral issues are also associated with FI. A longitudinal cohort study of young children found that growing up in food insecure households increased the likelihood of persistent symptoms of hyperactivity and inattention [94]. Recent findings suggest that food insecure students bully others and are victims of bullying more frequently than food secure students [95]. Finally, food insecure adolescents appear to have increased odds of engaging in "high risk behaviors," including smoking and drinking alcohol [96].

Children raised in food insecure households exhibit significantly lower levels of self-control during early childhood and higher levels of delinquency during late childhood than children raised in food secure households [97]. A longitudinal study of food insecure elementary school students found negative non-cognitive effects related to interpersonal relations, self-control, approaches to learning, and externalizing problem behaviors. The observed patterns indicated that early experiences were also predictive of subsequent, persistent effects even if a child's situation improved. Indeed, children experiencing FI in the 1st grade who were food secure by 3rd grade still showed evidence of impairments that persisted through 5th grade [98]. Longitudinal assessment of transitions into and out of household FI following the Great Recession found consistent negative impacts on externalizing behaviors, self-control, and interpersonal skills [99]. Separate research has suggested that household FI is negatively associated with social interaction ability among girls, affecting a child's ability to form friendships, express themselves, and maintain self-control [98, 100].

Academic and Developmental Health

The negative effects of FI and the importance of preventing exposure early in life is similarly evident in the academic and developmental health literature. A review conducted in 2017 demonstrated that household FI, even at marginal levels, is independently associated with a child's academic, behavioral, and emotional problems, stretching from infancy to adolescence, across western industrialized countries [101]. Early research using National Health and Nutrition Examination Survey (NHANES) III data and a concept similar to FI called "food insufficiency" (defined as "an inadequate amount of food intake due to a lack of resources") found that food insufficient 6–11 year-old children had significantly lower arithmetic scores than their food sufficient peers. They were also more likely to have repeated a grade, seen a psychologist, and had difficulty getting along with other children. Similarly, food insufficient teenagers were more likely to have seen a psychologist, been suspended from school, and had difficulty getting along with other children [47, 49]. Children in households with any signs of FI have been shown to receive lower test scores during the school year [102]. Moreover, FI in kindergarten predicts reduced academic achievement in math and reading over the subsequent 4-year period [103].

Conclusion

FI, as a key SDH, rarely travels alone. Often, food is the first resource to diminish in quantity or quality [39]. Those who are food insecure often experience other risks related to income, unemployment or underemployment, housing insecurity, energy insecurity, challenges with healthcare access, and structural discrimination [9, 104–106]. It is likely that these other determinants magnify the challenges faced by households dealing with FI, affecting health outcomes and perpetuating disparities. The twenty-first century clinician must see SDH as vital to the care they provide.

In the chapters that follow, we will provide additional insights into how clinicians can fill this role. We will outline how we can consistently recognize and respond to such risk factors (Chap. 2) with a range of interventions (Chap. 3) built with an eye toward population health (Chap. 4). Finally, we will introduce how interested parties can create action plans to address determinants like FI in a timely fashion (Chap. 5). We see such a path, toward action on FI and other SDH, as essential, one where the twenty-first century clinician supports their patients in their quest for the best possible outcomes.

References

1. Shonkoff JP, Garner AS, Siegel BS, Dobbins MI, Earls MF, Garner AS, et al. The lifelong effects of early childhood adversity and toxic stress. Pediatrics. 2012;129(1):e232–46.
2. Johnson SB, Riley AW, Granger DA, Riis J. The science of early life toxic stress for pediatric practice and advocacy. Pediatrics. 2013;131(2):319–27.
3. Marmot M, Friel S, Bell R, Houweling TAJ, Taylor S, Commission on Social Determinants of Health. Closing the gap in a generation: health equity through action on the social determinants of health. Lancet. 2008;372(9650):1661–9.
4. Galea S, Tracy M, Hoggatt KJ, Dimaggio C, Karpati A. Estimated deaths attributable to social factors in the United States. Am J Public Health. 2011;101(8):1456–65.
5. Anderson SA. Core indicators of nutritional state for difficult-to-sample populations. J Nutr. 1990;120(Suppl 11):1559–600.
6. Coleman-Jensen A, Rabbitt MP, Gregory CA, Singh A. Household Food Security in the United States in 2016. 2017 [cited 2017 Sep 18]. Available from: https://www.ers.usda.gov/webdocs/publications/84973/err-237.pdf?v=42979.
7. Messer E, Ross EM. Talking to patients about food insecurity. Nutr Clin Care. 2002;5(4):168–81.
8. Council NR. Food insecurity and hunger in the United States [Internet]. Washington, DC: National Academies Press; 2006. [cited 2017 Sep 18]. Available from: http://www.nap.edu/catalog/11578.
9. Alaimo K. Food insecurity in the United States. Top Clin Nutr. 2005;20(4):281.
10. Bickel G, Nord M, Price C, Hamilton W, Cook J. Measuring food security in the United States guide to measuring household food security revised 2000. [cited 2017 Sep 23]. Available from: http://www.fns.usda.gov/oane.
11. Radimer KL, Olson CM, Campbell CC. Development of indicators to assess hunger. J Nutr. 1990;120(Suppl):1544–8.
12. Radimer KL, Olson CM, Greene JC, Campbell CC, Habicht J-P. Understanding hunger and developing indicators to assess it in women and children. J Nutr Educ. 1992;24(1):36S–44S.
13. Hamelin AM, Habicht JP, Beaudry M. Food insecurity: consequences for the household and broader social implications. J Nutr. 1999;129(2S Suppl):525S–8S.
14. Hamelin A-M, Beaudry M, Habicht J-P. Characterization of household food insecurity in Québec: food and feelings. Soc Sci Med. 2002;54(1):119–32.
15. Jones AD, Ngure FM, Pelto G, Young SL. What are we assessing when we measure food security? A compendium and review of current metrics. Adv Nutr. 2013;4(5):481–505.

16. Cook JT, Black M, Chilton M, Cutts D, Ettinger de Cuba S, Heeren TC, et al. Are Food Insecurity's Health Impacts Underestimated in the U.S. Population? Marginal Food Security Also Predicts Adverse Health Outcomes in Young U.S. Children and Mothers. Adv Nutr An Int Rev J. 2013;4(1):51–61.
17. Coleman-Jensen A, Rabbitt MP, Gregory CA, Singh A. United States Department of Agriculture Statistical Supplement to Household Food Security in the United States in 2016. 2017 [cited 2017 Sep 24]. Available from: https://www.ers.usda.gov/webdocs/publications/84981/ap-077.pdf?v=42979.
18. Frongillo EA. Validation of measures of food insecurity and hunger. J Nutr. 1999;129(2S Suppl):506S–9S.
19. Map the Meal Gap, 2017: Highlights of Findings For Overall and Child Food Insecurity. [cited 2017 Sep 24]. Available from: http://www.feedingamerica.org/research/map-the-meal-gap/2015/2015-mapthemealgap-exec-summary.pdf.
20. National Research Council; Division of Behavioral and Social Sciences and Education; Institute of Medicine; Committee on National Statistics; Food and Nutrition Board. Research Opportunities Concerning the Causes and Consequences of Child Food Insecurity and Hunger [Internet]. Washington, D.C.: National Academies Press; 2013 [cited 2017 Sep 24]. Available from: http://www.nap.edu/catalog/18504.
21. Cohen B, Parry J, Yang K. Household Food Security in the United States, 1998 and 1999 Detailed Statistical Report. 2002 [cited 2017 Sep 24]. Available from: https://www.ers.usda.gov/webdocs/publications/43142/35929_efan02011fm.pdf?v=41528.
22. Nord M, Romig K. Hunger in the Summer. J Child Poverty. 2006;12(2):141–58.
23. Nord M, Kantor LS. Seasonal variation in food insecurity is associated with heating and cooling costs among low-income elderly Americans. J Nutr. 2006;136(11):2939–44.
24. Berkowitz SA, Seligman HK, Basu S. Impact of food insecurity and SNAP participation on healthcare utilization and expenditures. [cited 2017 Nov 17]. Available from: https://uknowledge.uky.edu/cgi/viewcontent.cgi?referer=https://www.google.com/&httpsredir=1&article=1105&context=ukcpr_papers.
25. Knowles M, Rabinowich J, De Cuba SE, Cutts DB, Chilton M, et al. "Do You Wanna Breathe or Eat?": Parent perspectives on child health consequences of food insecurity, trade-offs, and toxic stress. Matern Child Health J. 2016;20:25–32.
26. Wilde PE, Nord M, Zager RE. In longitudinal data from the survey of program dynamics, 16.9% of the U.S. population was exposed to household food insecurity in a 5-Year period. J Hunger Environ Nutr. 2010;5(3):380–98.
27. Ryu J-H, Bartfeld JS. Household food insecurity during childhood and subsequent health status: the early childhood longitudinal study—Kindergarten Cohort. Am J Public Health. 2012;102(11):e50–5.
28. Chilton M, Black MM, Berkowitz C, Casey PH, Cook J, Cutts D, et al. Food insecurity and risk of poor health among US-born children of immigrants. Am J Public Health. 2009;99(3):556–62.
29. Jyoti DF, Frongillo EA, Jones SJ. Food insecurity affects school children's academic performance, weight gain, and social skills. J Nutr. 2005;135(12):2831–9.
30. Chilton M, Chyatte M, Breaux J. The negative effects of poverty & food insecurity on child development. Indian J Med Res. 2007;126(4):262–72.
31. Sun J, Knowles M, Patel F, Frank DA, Heeren TC, Chilton M. Childhood adversity and adult reports of food insecurity among households with children. Am J Prev Med. 2016;50(5):561–72.
32. Fram MS, Frongillo EA, Jones SJ, Williams RC, Burke MP, DeLoach KP, et al. Children are aware of food insecurity and take responsibility for managing food resources. J Nutr. 2011;141(6):1114–9.
33. Semega JL, Fontenot KR, Kollar MA. Income and poverty in the United States: 2016. 2017 [cited 2017 Sep 26]. Available from: https://www.census.gov/content/dam/Census/library/publications/2017/demo/P60-259.pdf.

34. Weinfield NS, Mills WG, Institute U, Borger C, Gearing WM, Macaluso T, et al. Hunger in America 2014 National Report prepared for feeding America. 2014 [cited 2017 Nov 24]. Available from: http://help.feedingamerica.org/HungerInAmerica/ hunger-in-america-2014-full-report.pdf?s_src=W17BORGSC&s_referrer=google&s_ subsrc=http%3A%2F%2Fwww.feedingamerica.org%2Fresearch%2Fhunger-in-america%2F%3Freferrer%3Dhttps%3A%2F%2Fwww.google. com%2F&_ga=2.149471030.187319475.1511553130-1583801818.1511553130.

35. Burkhardt MC, Beck AF, Kahn RS, Klein MD. Are our babies hungry? Food insecurity among infants in urban clinics. Clin Pediatr (Phila). 2012;51(3):238–43.

36. Swanson JA, Olson CM, Miller EO, Lawrence FC. Rural mothers' use of formal programs and informal social supports to meet family food needs: a mixed methods study. J Fam Econ Iss. 2008;29(4):674–90.

37. Gundersen C, Kreider B, Pepper J. The economics of food insecurity in the United States. Appl Econ Perspect Policy. 2011;33(3):281–303.

38. Nord M, Brent CP. Food insecurity in higher income households. 2002 [cited 2017 Sep 26]. Available from: https://www.ers.usda.gov/webdocs/publications/43200/31163_ efan02016_002.pdf?v=41479.

39. Edin K, Lein L. Making ends meet: how single mothers survive welfare and low-wage work. New York: Russell Sage Foundation; 1997. 305 p.

40. Gundersen C, Ziliak JP. Childhood food insecurity in the U.S.: trends, causes, and policy options. Futur Child. 2014;24(2):1–19.

41. Coleman-Jensen A, McFall W, Nord M. Food Insecurity in Households With Children. 2013 [cited 2017 Sep 18];2010–1. Available from: http://www.ers.usda.gov.

42. McIntyre L, Glanville NT, Raine KD, Dayle JB, Anderson B, Battaglia N. Do low-income lone mothers compromise their nutrition to feed their children? CMAJ. 2003;168(6):686–91.

43. Nord M. Youth are less likely to be food insecure than adults in the same household. J Hunger Environ Nutr. 2013;8(2):146–63.

44. Connell CL, Lofton KL, Yadrick K, Rehner TA. Children's experiences of food insecurity can assist in understanding its effect on their well-being. J Nutr. 2005;135(7):1683–90.

45. Popkin SJ, Scott MM, Galvez M. Impossible choices: teens and food insecurity in America. 2016 [cited 2017 Sep 26]. Available from: https://www.urban.org/sites/default/files/alfresco/ publication-pdfs/2000914-Impossible-Choices-Teens-and-Food-Insecurity-in-America.pdf.

46. Coleman-Jensen A, McFall W, Nord M. Food insecurity in households with children: prevalence, severity, and household characteristics, 2010–11/Alisha Coleman-Jensen, William McFall, Mark Nord. [Internet]. 2013. (Economic Information Bulletin: number 113). Available from: http://proxygw.wrlc.org/login?url=http://search.ebscohost.com/login.aspx? direct=true&db=edsgpr&AN=gpr000903180&site=eds-live&scope=site&authtype=ip,uid& custid=s8987071.

47. Alaimo K, Olson CM, Frongillo EA. Food insufficiency and American school-aged children's cognitive, academic, and psychosocial development. Pediatrics. 2001;108(1):44–53.

48. Alaimo K, Olson CM, Frongillo EA. Family food insufficiency, but not low family income, is positively associated with dysthymia and suicide symptoms in adolescents. J Nutr. 2002;132(4):719–25.

49. Casey PH, Szeto KL, Robbins JM, Stuff JE, Connell C, Gossett JM, et al. Child health-related quality of life and household food security. Arch Pediatr Adolesc Med. 2005;159(1):51.

50. McLaughlin KA, Green JG, Alegría M, Jane Costello E, Gruber MJ, Sampson NA, et al. Food insecurity and mental disorders in a national sample of U.S. adolescents. J Am Acad Child Adolesc Psychiatry. 2012;51(12):1293–303.

51. Mary Morris L, Smith S, Davis J, Bloyd ND. The prevalence of food security and insecurity among Illinois University students. J Nutr Educ Behav. 2016;48:376–82.

52. Bruening M, Brennhofer S, van Woerden I, Todd M, Laska M. Factors related to the high rates of food insecurity among diverse, urban college freshmen. J Acad Nutr Diet. 2016 Sep;116(9):1450–7.

53. Hughes R, Serebryanikova I, Donaldson K, Leveritt M. Student food insecurity: the skeleton in the university closet. Nutr Diet. 2011;68(1):27–32.
54. Patton-López MM, López-Cevallos DF, Cancel-Tirado DI, Vazquez L. Prevalence and correlates of food insecurity among students attending a Midsize Rural University in Oregon. J Nutr Educ Behav. 2014;46(3):209–14.
55. Payne-Sturges DC, Tjaden A, Caldeira KM, Vincent KB, Arria AM. Student hunger on campus: food insecurity among college students and implications for academic institutions. Am J Health Promot. 2017;1:890117117719620. [Epub ahead of print].
56. Farahbakhsh J, Ball GDC, Farmer AP, Maximova K, Hanbazaza M, Willows ND. How do student clients of a university-based Food Bank Cope with food insecurity? Can J Diet Pract Res. 2015;76(4):200–3.
57. Maroto ME, Snelling A, Linck H. Food insecurity among community college students: prevalence and association with grade point average. Community Coll J Res Pract. 2015;39(6):515–26.
58. Hadley C, Patil CL, Nahayo D. Difficulty in the food environment and the experience of food insecurity among refugees resettled in the United States. Ecol Food Nutr. 2010;49(5):390–407.
59. Kalil A, Chen J-H. Mothers' citizenship status and household food insecurity among low-income children of immigrants. New Dir Child Adolesc Dev. 2008;2008(121):43–62.
60. Balistreri K, Hall W. Family structure, work patterns and time alloca-tions: potential mechanisms of food insecurity among children. 2012 [cited 2017 Sep 26]. Available from: http://uknowledge.uky.edu/cgi/viewcontent.cgi?article=1031&context=ukcpr_papers.
61. Cook J. Risk and protective factors associated with prevalence of VLFS in children among children of foreign-born mothers. [cited 2017 Sep 26]. Available from: http://uknowledge.uky.edu/cgi/viewcontent.cgi?article=1011&context=ukcpr_papers.
62. Hager ER, Quigg AM, Black MM, Coleman SM, Heeren T, Rose-Jacobs R, et al. Development and validity of a 2-item screen to identify families at risk for food insecurity. Pediatrics. 2010;126(1):e26 LP–e32.
63. Black MM, Drennen C, Gallego N, Coleman S, Frank DA. Household food insecurity is associated with children's health and developmental risks, but not with age-specific obesity and underweight. FASEB J. 2017;31(1 Supplement):791.17.
64. Cook JT, Frank DA, Berkowitz C, Black MM, Casey PH, Cutts DB, et al. Food insecurity is associated with adverse health outcomes among human infants and toddlers. J Nutr. 2004;134(6):1432–8.
65. Eicher-Miller HA, Mason AC, Weaver CM, McCabe GP, Boushey CJ. Food insecurity is associated with iron deficiency anemia in US adolescents. Am J Clin Nutr. 2009;90(5):1358–71.
66. Skalicky A, Meyers AF, Adams WG, Yang Z, Cook JT, Frank DA. Child food insecurity and iron deficiency anemia in low-income infants and toddlers in the United States. Matern Child Health J. 2006;10(2):177–85.
67. Kirkpatrick SI, McIntryre L, Potestio ML. Child hunger and long-term adverse consequences for health. Arch Pediatr Adolesc Med. 2010;164(8):754–62.
68. Chi DL, Masterson EE, Carle AC, Mancl LA, Coldwell SE. Socioeconomic status, food security, and dental caries in us children: Mediation analyses of data from the national health and nutrition examination survey, 2007–2008. Am J Public Health. 2014;104(5):860–4.
69. Hales CM, Carroll MD, Fryar CD, Ogden CL. Prevalence of obesity among adults and youth: United States, 2015–2016. NCHS Data Brief. 2017;288:1–8.
70. Frongillo EA, Bernal J. Understanding the coexistence of food insecurity and obesity. Curr Pediatr Rep. 2014;2(4):284–90.
71. Dietz WH. Does hunger cause obesity? Pediatrics. 1995;95(5):766–7.
72. Larson NI, Story MT, Nelson MC. Neighborhood environments. Am J Prev Med. 2009;36(1):74–81.e10.
73. Bruening M, MacLehose R, Loth K, Story M, Neumark-Sztainer D. Feeding a family in a recession: food insecurity among Minnesota parents. Am J Public Health. 2012;102(3):520–6.

74. Dammann K, Smith C. Food-related attitudes and behaviors at home, school, and restaurants: perspectives from racially diverse, urban, low-income 9- to 13-year-old children in Minnesota. J Nutr Educ Behav. 2010;42(6):389–97.
75. Scheier LM. What is the hunger-obesity paradox? J Am Diet Assoc. 2005;105(6):883–5.
76. Drewnowski A, Specter SE. Poverty and obesity: the role of energy density and energy costs. Am J Clin Nutr. 2004;79(1):6–16.
77. Kaur J, Lamb MM, Ogden CL. The association between food insecurity and obesity in children—The national health and nutrition examination survey. J Acad Nutr Diet. 2015;115(5):751–8.
78. Casey PH, Simpson PM, Gossett JM, Bogle ML, Champagne CM, Connell C, et al. The association of child and household food insecurity with childhood overweight status. Pediatrics. 2006;118(5):e1406–13.
79. Dubois L, Farmer A, Girard M, Porcherie M. Family food insufficiency is related to overweight among preschoolers. Soc Sci Med. 2006;63(6):1503–16.
80. Casey PH, Szeto K, Lensing S, Bogle M, Weber J. Children in food-insufficient, low-income families: prevalence, health, and nutrition status. Arch Pediatr Adolesc Med. 2001;155(4):508–14.
81. Rose D, Bodor JN. Household food insecurity and overweight status in young school children: results from the early childhood longitudinal study. Pediatrics. 2006;117(2):464–73.
82. Matheson DM, Varady J, Varady A, Killen JD. Household food security and nutritional status of Hispanic children in the fifth grade. Am J Clin Nutr. 2002;76(1):210–7.
83. Jiménez-Cruz A, Bacardí-Gascón M, Spindler AA. Obesity and hunger among Mexican-Indian migrant children on the US-Mexico border. Int J Obes Relat Metab Disord. 2003;27(6):740–7.
84. Gundersen C, Garasky S, Lohman BJ. Food insecurity is not associated with childhood obesity as assessed using multiple measures of obesity. J Nutr. 2009;139(6):1173–8.
85. Trapp CM, Burke G, Gorin AA, Wiley JF, Hernandez D, Crowell RE, et al. The relationship between dietary patterns, body mass index percentile, and household food security in young urban children. Child Obes. 2015;11(2):148–55.
86. Bhargava A, Jolliffe D, Howard LL. Socio-economic, behavioural and environmental factors predicted body weights and household food insecurity scores in the Early Childhood Longitudinal Study-Kindergarten. Br J Nutr. 2008;100(2):438–44.
87. Ma CT, Gee L, Kushel MB. Associations between housing instability and food insecurity with health care access in low-income children. Ambul Pediatr. 2008;8(1):50–7.
88. Palakshappa D, Khan S, Feudtner C, Fiks AG. Acute health care utilization among food-insecure children in primary care practices. J Health Care Poor Underserved. 2016;27(3):1143–58.
89. Lawson NR, Klein MD, Ollberding NJ, Wurster Ovalle V, Beck AF. The impact of infant well-child care compliance and social risks on emergency department utilization. Clin Pediatr (Phila). 2017;56(10):920–7.
90. Molcho M, Gabhainn SN, Kelly C, Friel S, Kelleher C. Food poverty and health among schoolchildren in Ireland: findings from the Health Behaviour in School-aged Children (HBSC) study. Public Health Nutr. 2007;10(4):364–70.
91. McIntyre L, Williams JVA, Lavorato DH, Patten S. Depression and suicide ideation in late adolescence and early adulthood are an outcome of child hunger. J Affect Disord. 2013;150(1):123–9.
92. McIntyre L, Wu X, Kwok C, Patten SB. The pervasive effect of youth self-report of hunger on depression over 6 years of follow up. Soc Psychiatry Psychiatr Epidemiol. 2017;52(5):537–47.
93. Stickley A, Leinsalu M. Childhood hunger and depressive symptoms in adulthood: findings from a population-based study. J Affect Disord. 2018;226:332–8.
94. Melchior M, Chastang J-F, Falissard B, Dric C, Ra G, Tremblay RE, et al. Food insecurity and children's mental health: a prospective birth cohort study. PLoS One. 2012;7(12):e52615.
95. Edwards OW, Taub GE. Children and youth perceptions of family food insecurity and bullying. Sch Ment Heal. 2017;9(3):263–72.

96. Robson SM, Lozano AJ, Papas M, Patterson F. Food insecurity and cardiometabolic risk factors in adolescents. Prev Chronic Dis. 2017;14:170222.
97. Jackson DB, Newsome J, Vaughn MG, Johnson KR. Considering the role of food insecurity in low self-control and early delinquency. J Crim Justice. 14 July 2017 Jul [Epub ahead of print].
98. Howard LL. Does food insecurity at home affect non-cognitive performance at school? A longitudinal analysis of elementary student classroom behavior. Econ Educ Rev. 2010;30:157–76.
99. Kimbro RT, Denney JT. Transitions into food insecurity associated with behavioral problems and worse overall health among children. Health Aff (Millwood). 2015;34(11):1949–55.
100. Stormer, A, Harrison GG. Does household food security affect cognitive and social development of Kindergartners? – Policy file index – ProQuest [Internet]. Institute for Research on Poverty. 2003 [cited 2017 Nov 25]. Available from: https://proxy.library.upenn.edu:7450/policyfile/docview/1820849651.
101. Shankar P, Chung R, Frank DA. Association of food insecurity with children's behavioral, emotional, and academic outcomes: a systematic review. J Dev Behav Pediatr. 2017;38(2):135–50.
102. Winicki J, Jemison K. Food insecurity and hunger in the Kindergarten classroom: its effect on learning and growth. Contemp Econ Policy. 2003;21(2):145–57.
103. Joyti DF, Frongillo EA, Jones SJ. Food insecurity affects school children's academic performance, weight gain, and social skills. J Nutr. 2005;135:2891–39.
104. Gundersen C. Measuring the extent, depth, and severity of food insecurity: an application to American Indians in the USA. J Popul Econ. 2008;21(1):191–215.
105. Gordon C, Purciel-Hill M, Ghai NR, Kaufman L, Graham R, Van Wye G. Measuring food deserts in New York City's low-income neighborhoods. Health Place. 2011;17(2):696–700.
106. Coleman-Jensen AJ. Working for peanuts: nonstandard work and food insecurity across household structure. J Fam Econ Iss. 2011;32(1):84–97.

Chapter 2
Impacting Food Insecurity Through the Use of Screening Tools and Training

Kofi Essel, Baraka D. Floyd, and Melissa Klein

Abbreviations

AAP   American Academy of Pediatrics
EHR   Electronic Health Record
FI   Food Insecurity
FRAC   Food Research & Action Center
HFSSM   Household Food Security Survey Module
HVS   Hunger Vital Sign
SDH   Social Determinants of Health
US   United States

Aims

1. Examine individual screening tools available to assess for food insecurity in clinical settings
2. Describe comprehensive social determinants screening tools that incorporate food insecurity screening
3. Explore methods to train clinicians on food insecurity screening and management

Food insecurity (FI) is a critical social determinant, as the lack of food is associated with a variety of deleterious outcomes, including psychosocial, physical, and

K. Essel (✉)
Children's National Health System, The George Washington University,
School of Medicine & Health Sciences, Washington, DC, USA
e-mail: kessel@childrensnational.org

B. D. Floyd
Stanford School of Medicine, Stanford, CA, USA

M. Klein
Cincinnati Children's Hospital Medical Center and University of Cincinnati College of Medicine,
Cincinnati, OH, USA

© The Author(s) 2018   23
H. B. Kersten et al. (eds.), *Identifying and Addressing Childhood Food
Insecurity in Healthcare and Community Settings*, SpringerBriefs in Public
Health, https://doi.org/10.1007/978-3-319-76048-3_2

developmental sequelae in children (Review Chap. 1 for details) [1]. Although children are often spared from the inadequate food supply, as parents prioritize food for children, they still may experience an extended burden of household psychosocial risk [2–6]. The constant preoccupation with food in adults may lead to decreased "cognitive bandwidth" leading to an inability to shift focus to other necessary responsibilities, like time and attention to themselves and their children, that allow the entire household to function effectively [7–9].

FI affects all populations and is a social determinant that clinicians will encounter clinically. In addition, FI is not consistently and reliably associated with anthropometric, laboratory, or clinical findings, and therefore may be described as invisible, requiring deliberate, specific screening [10]. In 2015, the American Academy of Pediatrics (AAP) created its first policy statement on FI, encouraging providers to screen for and intervene on behalf of families to address FI in their clinical settings [11]. This policy statement encouraged providers to screen at scheduled routine healthcare maintenance visits, advocated for programs and policies that end childhood FI, and supported use of a specific screening tool called the "Hunger Vital Sign" [11].

An increasing number of studies have examined pediatric provider screening practices [12–16]. FI screening is difficult and new for many providers; in fact, historically, only 11–15% of pediatric providers routinely screened [12, 13, 16]. Challenges associated with screening include time constraints, unknown or lack of resources, limited knowledge, personal discomfort and concerns about families' responses [12–14, 16, 17]. In addition, since most physicians were not raised in poverty, they cannot rely on their own past experiences, thus formal education, related to both poverty and screening, is necessary [14, 15, 18–20].

Effective screening in clinical practice involves utilizing specific screening tools in conjunction with meaningful interventions [21–23]. FI screening tools must balance their ability to detect food insecure families (i.e. high sensitivity) without being a burden to clinical work flow (i.e. rapidly administered, easily interpretable) [11, 24, 25]. A variety of FI screening tools have been used in research and clinical settings. The next section will outline some of the tools; a more extensive list along with the benefits and challenges to use in clinical practice are described in Table 2.1.

The 18-item Household Food Security Survey Module (HFSSM) is the gold standard screener collected by the United States (US) Census Bureau's Current Population Survey [26]. The survey tool was developed by an expert panel and collects household level information related to a lack of economic resources [26–29]. Since the HFSSM describes the household, this measure is unable to measure hunger, a measure of an individual's sensation or discomfort. The HFSSM has mainly been used in research studies to provide an accurate assessment of household food security or to evaluate severity of household food security [10, 30, 31]. An expert panel decided hunger should be measured distinctly from *household* FI, thus other screening tools may be necessary [29].

The Hunger Vital Sign (HVS) is a 2 question FI screener developed directly from the 18-item HFSSM [10, 11, 32]. This screen has been validated in clinical

Table 2.1 Food Insecurity Screeners and their positive and negative attributes in clinical practice

Name of screening tool	Pros for clinical use	Cons for clinical use	Sensitivity/specificity households w/ children
18-item Household Food Security Survey Module (HFSSM) [27–29]	• US gold standard: Most accurate assessment of household food security • Measures 3 components of food insecurity (see Chap. 1) • Measures severity and depth of food insecurity • Able to detect food insecurity amongst children	• Does not effectively measure all components of FI (see Chap. 1) • Long and complicated	• Gold standard
6-item Short form of the food security survey module [28, 76, 77]	• Adapted from 18-item HFSSM • Assesses severity and depth of household food security • Basic insight into children's experiences • Reduced survey response burden	• No child FI specific questions • May still be burdensome in clinical practice	• Sensitivity: 85.9% • Specificity: 99.5%
2-item Hunger vital sign [10, 30]	• Most widely used screening tool in US clinical settings • Incorporated in multiple comprehensive screeners (see Table 2.2) • Accepted by many clinical practices and national organizations [11, 24, 78] • Brief and efficient screening	• FI severity is not measured • No child FI specific questions	• Sensitivity: 97% • Specificity: 83%
1-item Food questionnaire from Canada [79]	• One or both questions can be used • Screener is tailored to indicate FI in children within a household	• The tool was manipulated extensively decreasing the validity • Generalizability may be limited due to validation in a unique population	• Sensitivity: 88.4–93% • Specificity: 93.4–97.3%
1-item Hunger screening question by Kleinman [35]	• Brief and efficient screenings in clinical setting	• Limited ability in detecting less severe food insecurity • Screening tool asks about the last month's experience, rather than 12 months, so may not capture the data needed to assess the families need • High misclassification rate • Limited ability to detect the depth of FI severity	• Sensitivity: 83% • Specificity: 80%

(continued)

Table 2.1 (continued)

Name of screening tool	Pros for clinical use	Cons for clinical use	Sensitivity/specificity households w/ children
Screeners to identify food insecurity in children			
8-item Children's food security scale [6, 80]	• Adapted from 18-item HFSSM (questions 11–18) • Most accurate tool to determine food security *among* children in a household • Has the ability to assess the full range of household food security among children	• Does not allow for household level data, only the experiences of children in the household • May be too long and complex for clinical use	• Unavailable
9-item Child food security survey module (self-administered) [36, 37]	• Distinguishes three layers of food security severity in children • Allows clinical teams to understand food insecurity through the experience of teenage youth • Enhanced recognition of the child's experience may allow for additional resources • May be administered on a web based platform, reported as more comfortable for teens	• Limited ability to correctly identify a child with very low FI (sensitivity 77%) • May be too long and complex for clinical use	• Sensitivity: 89% • Specificity: 93%
2-item Hunger vital sign (self-administered) [38]	• Efficient 2 question screener • Allows clinical teams to understand food insecurity through the teenager's experience • Enhanced recognition of the child's experience may allow for added/different resources • May be administered on a web based platform	• Since questions related to income, adolescents may be less aware, limiting the accuracy • May need a more extensive questionnaire if patient answers with a positive response	• Sensitivity: 88.5% • Specificity: 84.1%

settings demonstrating very high sensitivity (97%) and relatively high specificity (83%) [10]. Compared with the 18-item HFSSM, the HVS has shown strong accuracy amongst adults with young children, older children and adolescents, and other high risk groups (households with children, elderly, ethnic minorities, immigrant families, individuals with disability, or income <200% of the federal poverty line) [10, 30]. Due to its brevity and high performance, it has been adopted in many clinical and research settings [14, 15, 39]. The original HVS was created with a 3 point Likert response ("Often True", "Sometimes True", or "Never True") where both "Often True" and "Sometimes True" were considered an affirmative response. Advocates and researchers recommended switching to a dichotomous response ("Yes" or "No") to simplify face-to-face screening [11, 15]. However, the dichotomous response can create a challenge for some families and has been linked with reducing the number of affirmative responses by up to 25% as compared to the complete HVS [33]. For example, families may already be concerned that a doctor may call child protective services for child neglect if they admit to FI [15, 25, 34]. The "sometimes true" response may serve as a buffer zone for families, while at the same time, allowing them to indicate a need to the provider [33].

The Single-Question Hunger Screening Tool was one of the earliest tools created to detect hunger in the clinical setting. This tool was specifically developed to screen for a family's experience of hunger [35]. In 2004, compared to the full 18-item HFSSM, the single question screener demonstrated 83% sensitivity and 80% specificity to identify FI [35]. This survey was designed for the prior definition of FI (with/without hunger) compared to the more recent FI definition (low/very low food security) [26, 28].

In order to better measure the lived experience of a child in a food insecure household, there are two available tools, the Child Food Security Survey Module and Hunger Vital Sign, that may be self-administered or asked to children over the age of 12 years [36–38].

FI Screening Embedded Within a Broader Social Risk Screening Tool

As FI often coexists with other social risks, more comprehensive social risk screening tools may be beneficial. Since a gold standard social screening tool has not been identified, organizations and clinical practices have created social risk screeners tailored to their communities incorporating available validated questions. There are a variety of more comprehensive social risk screening tools that can be incorporated into clinical practice. Table 2.2 details a few commonly used social risk screeners that contain specific FI questions.

Table 2.2 Social risk screening tools

Screening tool	Domains covered	Food security/ access questions used
AHC HRSN (Accountable Health Communities Health Related Social Needs) Tool [78] https://innovation.cms.gov/ initiatives/ahcm	• Housing instability • Food insecurity • Transportation difficulties • Utility assistance needs • Interpersonal safety concerns	• Hunger vital sign(slightly modified)[a] "1. Within the past 12 months, you worried that your food would run out before you got money to buy more 2. Within the past 12 months, the food you bought just didn't last and you didn't have money to get more." • *Response: Often True, Sometimes True, Never True*
WE-CARE (Well-child Care Visit, Evaluation, Community Resources, Advocacy, Referral, Education) [16, 43] www.pediatrics.org/cgi/ doi/10.1542/peds.2007–0398	• Education • Employment • Smoking/drug/alcohol abuse • Depression • Domestic violence • Child care • Housing • Food supply	• "Do you need help in getting food by the end of the month?" • *Response: Yes, No,* • *–If yes, would you like help with this?* • *Yes, No, Maybe Later*
Health Leads https://healthleadsusa.org/ tools-item/ health-leads-screening-toolkit/	• Food insecurity • Housing instability • Utility needs • Financial resource strain • Transportation • Exposure to violence • Sociodemographic information	• Question #6 from HFSSM • "In the last 12 months, did you ever eat less than you felt you should because there wasn't enough money for food?" • *Response: Yes or No*
Survey of Wellbeing of Young Children (SWYC) https://www.floatinghospital.org/ The-Survey-of-Wellbeing-of-Young-Children/Overview.aspx	**Family questions domains:** • Parental depression • Parental discord • Substance abuse • Food insecurity • Parent's concerns about the child's behavior/ learning/ • Development	• One question hunger Screener[a] [31] • "In the past month, was there any day when you or anyone in your family went hungry because you did not have enough money for food?" • *Response:* • *Yes, No*
I-HELLP (Income, Housing, Education, Legal Status, Literacy, Personal Safety) [81] https://www.aap.org/en-us/ Documents/IHELLPPocketCard. pdf	• Income • Housing • Education • Legal status • Literacy • Personal safety	• "Do you ever have a time when you don't have enough food? Do you have WIC? Food stamps?" • *Response:* • *Yes, No*

(continued)

Table 2.2 (continued)

Screening tool	Domains covered	Food security/access questions used
SEEK (Safe Environment for Every Kid) https://www.seekwellbeing.org/the-seek-parent-questionnaire-	• Parental depression • Parental substance abuse • Harsh punishment • Major parental stress • Intimate partner violence • Food insecurity	• Hunger vital Sign[a] "1. In the past 12 months, did you worry that your food would run out before you could buy more? 2. In the past 12 months, did the food you bought just not last and you didn't have money to get more?" • *Response:* • *Yes, No*

[a]Indicates clinically validated screening tool

FI Screening in Clinical Practice

General Principles

Both clinicians and families may express unease with FI screening due to the sensitive nature of these questions [13, 15, 24]. Similar to asking about other psychosocial issues, clinicians must learn about the root causes of FI, the family perspective and resources to address FI, so they can effectively and empathetically screen. Parents have reported feelings of shame, guilt, and frustration when they are unable to provide enough food for their families, have concerns that clinicians would consider them neglectful and as mentioned previously, may notify child protective services if they admit to FI [15, 25, 34]. As practices transition to addressing the entire family's social risks, it may be beneficial to provide information indicating that questions are asked universally and that the responses will be used to help the family and not penalize them [9, 14, 22, 25]. This may create a safe atmosphere for families to disclose [25].

Frequency

The ideal frequency of FI screening has not been established; however, there have been several different recommendations. Since FI is invisible and often not detected by growth parameters, experts recommend routine, universal screening, despite the additional demand on time [40]. Universal screening can decrease effects of implicit bias [22, 41, 42] and more reliably identify families in need than provider driven screening [43–45]. In addition, universal screening decreases stigma and isolation for families with FI concerns.

Garg & Dworkin provide specific recommendations of screening during initial visits, all visits in the first 6 months of life, annually during routine well-child visits and whenever problems are detected [21]. The Food Research & Action Center (FRAC), a national anti-hunger policy organization, and the AAP proposed a toolkit for pediatricians to screen and intervene for FI. The expert panel proposed screening all patients at all visits due to the hidden and cyclical nature of FI, but in cases where providers must prioritize, screening was recommended at particular visits: (1) Routine well-child care; (2) Nutrition-related concerns (e.g., diabetes, obesity, food allergies); (3) Emergency medicine visits; (4) Hospital admissions; (5) Newborns prior to discharge; (6) As indicated during any other visit (e.g., parent mentions recent job loss, child with anemia or behavioral problems, patient requires a special diet or expensive medication) [24].

Implementing a Screening Process

Once the clinical team decides which FI screening tool to use, the next decision is how the screening will be implemented. A team based approach, including clinicians, trainees, nurses, medical assistants, social workers, and community health workers may be most effective for FI screening [24]. To maximize success, training should specify each individual's role on the team, related to their area of expertise. Screening that maximizes use of downtime during the visit (i.e. waiting room or waiting time in the examination room) may improve potential for success by allowing parents the time to complete the screener without increasing the visit length. It is important to remember that children above the age of 12 years old may be screened directly using one of the pediatric FI screening tools (e.g. 9-item Child Food Security Module, Hunger Vital Sign). In addition, completion of a screening tool prior to the visit allows the clinician to review the responses and plan an intervention with the family [14, 21, 46].

Written screening tools are accepted by patients, families and clinicians. Ideally, these are quickly reviewed during the visit and used to plan interventions in a family-centered fashion [47]. These screeners must be provided in the patient's preferred language, administered in a safe and private area and ideally entered into the electronic health record (EHR). Additional procedures need to be in place for patients and families with low literacy levels to obtain accurate responses.

Computer Based Self-Administered Screening Tools are typically accessed by a waiting room kiosk, clinic based tablet or personalized electronic device. They have similar drawbacks (language, literacy, privacy) to paper-based screeners, however, screen protectors may allow for added privacy [17]. These tools may provide for cost savings, but may also limit connection between clinician and families [48]. Electronic screeners have demonstrated increased transparency in responses and less limitation by social desirability bias compared to face-to-face screening [48, 49]. In general, with issues of increased sensitivity, written and computer based screeners may provide the most safety and protection for families [25, 48].

Face-to-Face Screening is another method used to identify social risks, including FI. Verbal screening may allow for increased connection between clinicians and families, but may increase shame and underestimate concern due to social desirability bias [48, 50]. With older children present, parents may feel even less comfortable discussing the family's food security status [25, 51, 52]. Although verbal screening may seem the most efficient for screening adolescents when parents leave the examination room, adolescents have reported that they may prefer electronic or computer based screening [65]. Verbal screening also offers the most challenge with maintaining fidelity of questions as questioning style may change, shorten or lengthen based on memory recall or personal biases that one may carry [53, 54]. Verbal screeners are a safe way of screening when identifying one or few SDH but may not be the most effective or efficient when screening for multiple social risks.

Documentation

Incorporation of responses to screening questions into the EHR can greatly increase the feasibility and likelihood of routine screening [48, 55, 56]. After determining the screening tool and method that works best in the clinical setting, it is important to determine documentation practice. An Institute of Medicine report recommended documentation of food security, one component of social risk, in the EHR; with nearly universal use of EHRs in medical practices, this is rapidly becoming possible [57, 58]. Standardized documentation can systematically capture screening results and measure changes over time for an individual patient or population. Refer to Chap. 5 for additional details on in-clinic and community resources.

Training in Social Determinants, Including Food Insecurity

When developing a social determinants of health curriculum, it is important to consider several principles of adult learning theory. Since adult learners build on previous lived experience, it is critical to recognize their prior knowledge and experiences [59, 60] that may shape biases and impact learning. Since many medical trainees were not raised in poverty [61], they have not personally experienced [62] many of the social risks in their patients' lives, including FI, making it difficult to relate to their patients' experiences. The often privileged, discordant backgrounds of providers can make tackling questions related to socioeconomic status difficult, contribute to their discomfort screening, and limit their awareness of needs or willingness to screen for and address FI. Thus, creating experiences that simulate patients' lived experiences, the so-called "walk in your shoes" experiences, may be beneficial.

Essential components of FI curricula should include: (1) Definitions and Epidemiology; (2) Physiologic and Psychosocial Impact; (3) Screening Methods and Strategies; (4) Intervention Strategies and Community Resources; and (5) Associated Social Risks [63–71]. To maximize effectiveness, it is ideal to develop and implement curricula that incorporate a variety of learning modalities and tasks to appeal to different learning styles. For example, to fully grasp a concept, learners could be expected to complete pre-reading, participate in a case based, interactive session that allows them to apply their new knowledge and then implement a small project in the continuity clinic. This provides learning opportunities for visual, aural, reflective and kinesthetic learners [72, 73]. This deliberate connection and application to real-life, clinical settings are essential for meaningful learning [59, 74]. However, curriculum design always needs to remain cognizant of the barriers (i.e. lack of time, confidence and motivation [62]) that may be unique to medical trainees.

Existing SDH Curricula that Include FI

As one considers training clinicians to address FI, there are several publically available curricula that have been created for medical students or resident and attending physicians. Here, we briefly describe the aim and target audience for a few curricula, but acknowledge these are only samples and not an exhaustive list. In Table 2.3, we highlight different educational strategies and learning activities in these curricula.

The Academic Pediatric Associations' US Child Poverty Curriculum is publically available on the AAP Community Pediatrics Training Initiative website (https://www.aap.org/en-us/advocacy-and-policy/aap-health-initiatives/CPTI/Pages/U-S-Child-Poverty-Curriculum.aspx) [63]. This curriculum, created for Pediatric residents and medical students addresses (1) Epidemiology of Child Poverty; (2) Social Determinants of Health; (3) Biomedical Influences of Poverty; and (4) Taking Action to Address Child Poverty [64]. Designed by pediatricians, educators and health science researchers across the US, this curriculum can be implemented in different settings (i.e. community pediatric rotation, continuity clinic) and formats (i.e. 60-min sessions, half day retreats). The online material includes pre-work, presentations and suggested interactive activities for each module. In addition, there is an instructor guide to permit presentation by faculty who do not consider themselves SDH experts [65].

Inquiring about FI and other issues related to poverty has not been traditionally taught in medical school, thus many clinicians may benefit from training on screening families. We encourage all overarching SDH curricula include a component related to effective screening. At Cincinnati Children's Hospital, a curriculum composed of a series of videos was developed to help trainees increase both confidence and competence in SDH screening. The impact of parent voice is increasingly recognized as critical; thus, some curricula focus on including the patients' perspective in either the education or evaluation component. In the Cincinnati Children's video curriculum, short videos with a family describing the effect of the SDH on their family and the impact of screening and intervention have proven critical for learners. The curriculum also includes accessing in-clinic and community resources that can help mitigate these SDH [66].

Table 2.3 Educational modalities utilized in selected SDH curricula

Teaching strategy	Description	Pros	Cons	Example curricula
• Didactic presentation	• Lecturer delivers content to learners	• Lecturer reliably delivers specific information • Ability to deliver to larger number of learners • Audience response systems: • Strategy to increase engagement among a large group of learners [74]	• Passive learning • Impact depends teacher's effectiveness • May lack incorporation of learners' experiences and application to specific clinical setting	• US child poverty curriculum [64] • Health scholars program [68]
• Use of video/movie	• Video or movie used as teaching tool • Use of 360 video can provide a realistic view that simulates presence	• Ability to share patient voice • Hearing parent or patient story can be more impactful • Employs cycle of experience	• Needs to be used as a learning tool in a larger curriculum. • In absence of facilitation and context, learner may not connect to clinical setting	• Cincinnati Children's video trigger curriculum [61] • US child poverty curriculum [64]
• Shadowing	• Learner observes clinician practicing the desired skills	• Opportunity for experiential learning • Train in the actual clinical or community site	• Learner needs to be primed to be an active learner • Teacher needs skills to promote active learning with application	• Health scholars program [68]
• Flipped classroom [82]	• Learners review material prior to session and apply the knowledge in a group setting	• Allows students to be actively involved in thinking through common problems/formulate solutions • Self-assessment of learners' knowledge identifies gaps for focused facilitation • Utilizes often sparse teaching time for application of concepts, rather than knowledge transfer	• Learners need to review the material prior to the session • Weak evidence of efficacy for gaining knowledge [82]	• US child poverty curriculum [64] • AAP poverty statement [83] teaching session-Stanford community pediatrics rotation

(continued)

Table 2.3 (continued)

Teaching strategy	Description	Pros	Cons	Example curricula
• Practice based learning	• Learning in the context of direct clinical care	• Requires learner's engagement in material • Allows learners to apply simple concepts immediately	• Errors in application can have negative effects on families • Preceptor supervision and time management can be barrier • Requires significant instructor time and commitment to ensure mentorship and application	• OHSU child advocacy and community health [67] • Cincinnati Children's Geomedicine curriculum [75] • Boston combined residency program community health and advocacy rotation [71]
• Immersion	• Act of connecting learner to environment to learn perspective of patients and community members	• Provides realistic experience of communities for learners to build upon • Capitalizes on changing attitudes through experience of seeing another's perspective (i.e. walk in someone else's shoes)	• Difficult to coordinate due to limited time of both learner and community member • Needs to include time for facilitation, reflection and context to maximize learning impact • Risk of potential negative emotional response and safety concerns	• OHSU child advocacy and community health [67] • Health scholars program [68] • Cincinnati Children's surviving poverty series [84, 85]
• Spiral curriculum	• Iterative review of topics to deepen understanding	• Allows learners to build on prior experiences • Balances increasing challenges for learners at each stage with preventing frustration	• Requires attention to matching learning tasks to expected competency	• Cincinnati Children's Geomedicine curriculum [75] • Boston combined residency program community health and advocacy rotation [71]

Since many clinicians may not recognize the pervasiveness and impact of poverty, residency programs and medical schools have created a variety of educational experiences that vary in duration, content and format. Some programs have implemented longitudinal experiences on poverty, SDH and child health. Oregon Health Sciences University Doernbecher Children's Project REACH (Resident Experience in Advocating for Children's Health) is one example. Residents in this program participate in didactic lectures and experiential learning that include practicing in local safety net clinics, engaging with community agencies, and exploring the neighborhoods where patient's live. Additionally, residents complete group advocacy projects [67]. The Health Scholars Program, a longitudinal curriculum for undergraduate medical students at Temple University, University of Pennsylvania, Drexel University, Jefferson Medical College, and Philadelphia College of Osteopathic Medicine, aims to increase the number of physicians who will care for patients in underserved communities. This curriculum combines didactics with critical reflection and service in a community clinic [68].

Other pediatric residency programs have instituted advocacy or community pediatrics block rotations to provide dedicated, focused training on poverty, the SDH, including FI, and their impact on child health and well-being. Although these rotations may vary in structure and focus, there has been an increasing effort to increase trainees' recognition of the importance of neighborhood and patient context on health [69]. For example, Cincinnati Children's includes a spiral Geomedicine curriculum. The first-year residents have an experiential learning activity to introduce them to one impoverished neighborhood near the hospital. Residents connect the information they learn from community partners and families to health outcomes. As upper level residents, there are additional interactive, facilitated sessions that provide information on other impoverished neighborhoods and readily accessible websites during routine visits to aid families combating many of the SDH, including FI [70, 75]. The Boston Combined Residency program also has a neighborhood based curriculum that includes a community tour, multidisciplinary didactic session, and self-directed learning experience to explore local resources [71].

Summary

FI screening is an important part of clinical care, and begins with choosing the best screening tool for the clinical setting. Multidisciplinary clinical teams should be trained on FI screening, due to the complexity of detection and intervention. Medical students and residents will likely need training on screening, social risks and in-clinic and community resources. Curricula, with a variety of learning activities, should be implemented after reviewing currently available curricula and resources.

References

1. Coleman-Jensen A, McFall W, Nord M. Food insecurity in households with children. 2013 [cited 2017 Sep 18];2010–1. Available from: www.ers.usda.gov.
2. Chilton M, Black MM, Berkowitz C, Casey PH, Cook J, Cutts D, et al. Food insecurity and risk of poor health among US-born children of immigrants. [cited 2017 Sep 26]. Available from: https://www.ncbi.nlm.nih.gov/pmc/articles/PMC2661461/pdf/556.pdf.
3. Chilton M, Chyatte M, Breaux J. The negative effects of poverty & food insecurity on child development. Indian J Med Res [Internet]. 2007 Oct [cited 2017 Sep 28];126(4):262–72. Available from: http://www.ncbi.nlm.nih.gov/pubmed/18032801.
4. Sun J, Knowles M, Patel F, Frank DA, Heeren TC, Chilton M. Childhood adversity and adult reports of food insecurity among households with children. Am J Prev Med [Internet]. 2016 May [cited 2017 Sep 28];50(5):561–72. Available from: http://www.ncbi.nlm.nih.gov/pubmed/26596189.
5. Jyoti DF, Frongillo EA, Jones SJ. Food insecurity affects school children's academic performance, weight gain, and social skills. J Nutr [Internet]. 2005 Dec [cited 2017 Sep 28];135(12):2831–9. Available from: http://www.ncbi.nlm.nih.gov/pubmed/16317128.
6. Nord M, Bickel G. Measuring children's food security in U.S. households, 1995–99. US Households [Internet]. [cited 2017 Oct 13];1995–9. Available from: https://www.ers.usda.gov/webdocs/publications/46613/31444_fanrr25_002.pdf?v=41479.
7. National Academies of Sciences E and M. Meeting the dietary needs of older adults [Internet]. Rogers AB, Oria M, editors. Washington, DC: National Academies Press; 2016 [cited 2017 Oct 8]. Available from: http://www.nap.edu/catalog/23496.
8. Berkowitz SA, Seligman HK, Basu S. Impact of food insecurity and SNAP participation on healthcare utilization and expenditures. [cited 2017 Oct 8]. Available from: http://uknowledge.uky.edu/cgi/viewcontent.cgi?article=1105&context=ukcpr_papers.
9. Messer E, Ross EM, Ldn. Talking to patients about food insecurity. Nutr Clin Care [Internet]. 2002 Aug;5(4):168–81. Available from: http://10.4.22/j.1523-5408.2002.00303.x.
10. Hager ER, Quigg AM, Black MM, Coleman SM, Heeren T, Rose-Jacobs R, et al. Development and validity of a 2-item screen to identify families at risk for food insecurity. Pediatrics [Internet]. 2010 Jul 1;126(1):e26 LP–e32. Available from: http://pediatrics.aappublications.org/content/126/1/e26.abstract.
11. Promoting Food Security for All Children. Pediatrics [Internet]. 2015 Nov;136(5):e1431–8. Available from: http://proxygw.wrlc.org/login?url=http://search.ebscohost.com/login.aspx?direct=true&db=mdc&AN=26498462&site=eds-live&scope=site&authtype=ip,uid&custid=s8987071.
12. Hoisington AT, Braverman MT, Hargunani DE, Adams EJ, Alto CL. Health care providers' attention to food insecurity in households with children. Prev Med (Baltim) [Internet]. 2012 Sep 1;55:219–22. Available from: http://10.3.248/j.ypmed.2012.06.007.
13. Barnidge E, LaBarge G, Krupsky K, Arthur J. Screening for food insecurity in pediatric clinical settings: opportunities and barriers. J Community Health [Internet]. 2017 Aug 4. Available from: http://proxygw.wrlc.org/login?url=http://search.ebscohost.com/login.aspx?direct=true&db=mdc&AN=27492774&site=eds-live&scope=site&authtype=ip,uid&custid=s8987071.
14. Palakshappa D, Vasan A, Khan S, Seifu L, Feudtner C, Fiks AG. Clinicians' perceptions of screening for food insecurity in suburban pediatric practice. Pediatrics [Internet]. 2017 Jul 20 [cited 2017 Oct 8];140(1):e20170319. Available from: http://www.ncbi.nlm.nih.gov/pubmed/28634247.
15. Burkhardt MC, Beck AF, Conway PH, Kahn RS, Klein MD. Enhancing accurate identification of food insecurity using quality-improvement techniques. Pediatrics [Internet]. 2012 Feb 1 [cited 2017 Oct 8];129(2):e504–10. Available from: http://www.ncbi.nlm.nih.gov/pubmed/22250022.

16. Garg A, Butz AM, Dworkin PH, Lewis RA, Serwint JR. Screening for basic social needs at a medical home for low-income children. [cited 2017 Oct 8]. Available from: http://journals. sagepub.com/doi/pdf/10.1177/0009922808320602.

17. Fleegler EW, Lieu TA, Wise PH, Muret-Wagstaff S. Families' health-related social problems and missed referral opportunities. Pediatrics [Internet]. 2007 Jun 1 [cited 2017 Oct 10];119(6):e1332–41. Available from: http://www.ncbi.nlm.nih.gov/pubmed/17545363.

18. Wieland ML, Beckman TJ, Cha SS, Beebe TJ, McDonald FS, Underserved Care Curriculum Collaborative. Resident physicians' knowledge of underserved patients: a multi-institutional survey. Mayo Clin Proc [Internet]. 2010 Aug [cited 2017 Oct 8];85(8):728–33. Available from: http://www.ncbi.nlm.nih.gov/pubmed/20675511.

19. O'Toole JK, Burkhardt MC, Solan LG, Vaughn L, Klein MD. Resident confidence addressing social history. Clin Pediatr (Phila) [Internet]. 2012 Jul 7 [cited 2017 Oct 8];51(7):625–31. Available from: http://journals.sagepub.com/doi/10.1177/0009922812438081.

20. Knowles MS. Andragogy in action. San Francisco: Jossey-Bass; 1984. 444 p.

21. Garg A, Dworkin PH. Applying surveillance and screening to family psychosocial issues: implications for the medical home. J Dev Behav Pediatr [Internet]. 2011 Jun [cited 2016 Nov 16];32(5):418–26. Available from: http://content.wkhealth.com/linkback/openurl?sid=WKPT LP:landingpage&an=00004703-201106000-00010.

22. Chung EK, Siegel BS, Garg A, Conroy K, Gross RS, Long DA, et al. Screening for social determinants of health among children and families living in poverty: a guide for clinicians. Curr Probl Pediatr Adolesc Health Care [Internet]. 2016 May [cited 2017 Oct 8];46(5):135–53. Available from: http://www.ncbi.nlm.nih.gov/pubmed/27101890.

23. Garg A, Boynton-Jarrett R, Dworkin PH. Avoiding the unintended consequences of screening for social determinants of health. JAMA [Internet]. 2016 Aug 23 [cited 2017 Oct 8];316(8):813. Available from: http://jama.jamanetwork.com/article.aspx?doi=10.1001/jama.2016.9282.

24. Addressing food insecurity: a toolkit for pediatricians. 2017 [cited 2017 Oct 9]. Available from: http://www.frac.org/wp-content/uploads/frac-aap-toolkit.pdf.

25. Palakshappa D, Doupnik S, Vasan A, Khan S, Seifu L, Feudtner C, et al. Suburban families' experience with food insecurity screening in primary care practices. Pediatrics [Internet]. 2017 Jul 20 [cited 2017 Oct 8];140(1):e20170320. Available from: http://www.ncbi.nlm.nih.gov/ pubmed/28634248.

26. Coleman-Jensen A, Rabbitt MP, Gregory CA, Singh A. Household food security in the United States in 2016. 2017 [cited 2017 Sep 18]. Available from: https://www.ers.usda.gov/webdocs/ publications/84973/err-237.pdf?v=42979.

27. Jones AD, Ngure FM, Pelto G, Young SL. What are we assessing when we measure food security? A compendium and review of current metrics. Adv Nutr [Internet]. 2013 Sep 1 [cited 2017 Sep 23];4(5):481–505. Available from: http://www.ncbi.nlm.nih.gov/pubmed/24038241.

28. Bickel G, Nord M, Price C, Hamilton W, Cook J. Measuring food security in the United States guide to measuring household food security revised 2000. [cited 2017 Sep 23]. Available from: http://www.fns.usda.gov/oane.

29. Council NR. Food insecurity and hunger in the United States [Internet]. Washington, DC: National Academies Press; 2006 [cited 2017 Sep 18]. Available from: http://www.nap.edu/ catalog/11578.

30. Gundersen C, Engelhard EE, Crumbaugh AS, Seligman HK. Brief assessment of food insecurity accurately identifies high-risk US adults. Public Health Nutr [Internet]. 2017 Jun 20 [cited 2017 Oct 8];20(8):1367–71. Available from: http://www.ncbi.nlm.nih.gov/pubmed/28215190.

31. Kleinman RE, Murphy JM, Wieneke KM, Desmond MS, Schiff A, Gapinski JA. Use of a single-question screening tool to detect hunger in families attending a neighborhood health center. Ambul Pediatr. 2007 Jul;7(4):278–84.

32. Goldman N, Sheward R, Ettinger de Cuba S, Black M, Sandel M, Cook J, et al. The hunger vital sign: a new standard of care for preventive health [Internet]. Children's Healthwatch Policy Action Brief. Boston; 2014 [cited 2018 Jan 3]. Available from: http://www.children- shealthwatch.org/wp-content/uploads/FINAL-Hunger-Vital-Sign-2-pager1.pdf.

33. Makelarski JA, Abramsohn E, Benjamin JH, Du S, Lindau ST. Diagnostic accuracy of two food insecurity screeners recommended for use in health care settings. Am J Public Health [Internet]. 2017 Nov [cited 2017 Dec 11];107(11):1812–7. Available from: http://www.ncbi.nlm.nih.gov/pubmed/28933929.
34. Gottlieb LM, Hessler D, Long D, Laves E, Burns AR, Amaya A, et al. Effects of social needs screening and in-person service navigation on child health. JAMA Pediatr [Internet]. 2016 Nov 7 [cited 2017 Oct 9];170(11):e162521. Available from: http://www.ncbi.nlm.nih.gov/pubmed/27599265.
35. Kleinman RE, Michael Murphy J, Little M, Pagano M, Wehler CA, et al. Hunger in children in the United States: potential behavioral and emotional correlates. [cited 2017 Oct 8]. Available from: http://pediatrics.aappublications.org/content/pediatrics/101/1/e3.full.pdf.
36. Connell CL, Nord M, Lofton KL, Yadrick K. Community and international nutrition food security of older children can be assessed using a standardized survey instrument 1. J Nutr [Internet]. 2004 [cited 2017 Oct 9];134:2566–72. Available from: http://jn.nutrition.org/content/134/10/2566.full.pdf.
37. Coleman-Jensen A, Nord M. Self-administered food security survey module for children ages 12 years and older. J Nutr [Internet]. 2004 [cited 2017 Oct 9];134(10):2566–72. Available from: https://www.ers.usda.gov/media/8283/youth2006.pdf.
38. Baer TE, Scherer EA, Fleegler EW, Hassan A. Food insecurity and the burden of health-related social problems in an urban youth population. J Adolesc Heal [Internet]. 2015 Dec [cited 2017 Oct 8];57(6):601–7. Available from: http://www.ncbi.nlm.nih.gov/pubmed/26592328.
39. Adams E, Hargunani D, Hoffmann L, Blaschke G, Helm J, Koehler A. Screening for food insecurity in pediatric primary care: a clinic's positive implementation experiences. J Health Care Poor Underserved [Internet]. 2017 [cited 2017 Oct 14];28(1):24–9. Available from: https://muse.jhu.edu/article/648742.
40. Fierman AH, Beck AF, Chung EK, Tschudy MM, Coker TR, Mistry KB, et al. Redesigning health care practices to address childhood poverty. Acad Pediatr [Internet]. 2016 Apr [cited 2017 Oct 10];16(3):S136–46. Available from: http://www.ncbi.nlm.nih.gov/pubmed/27044692.
41. Cheng TL, Emmanuel MA, Levy DJ, Jenkins RR. Child health disparities: what can a clinician do? [cited 2017 Oct 9]. Available from: http://pediatrics.aappublications.org/content/pediatrics/early/2015/10/06/peds.2014-4126.full.pdf.
42. Keller D, Jones N, Savageau JA, Cashman SB. Development of a brief questionnaire to identify families in need of legal advocacy to improve child health. Ambul Pediatr [Internet]. 2008 Jul [cited 2017 Oct 10];8(4):266–9. Available from: http://www.ncbi.nlm.nih.gov/pubmed/18644550.
43. Garg A, Toy S, Tripodis Y, Silverstein M, Freeman E. Addressing social determinants of health at well child care visits: a cluster RCT. Pediatrics [Internet]. 2015 Feb;135(2):e296–304. Available from: http://proxygw.wrlc.org/login?url=http://search.ebscohost.com/login.aspx?direct=true&db=mdc&AN=25560448&site=eds-live&scope=site&authtype=ip,uid&custid=s8987071.
44. Billioux A, Katherine V, Anthony S, Alley D. Standardized screening for health-related social needs in clinical settings the accountable health communities screening tool. Washington, DC: National Academy of Medicine; 2017.
45. Bikson K, McGuire J, Blue-Howells J, Seldin-Sommer L. Psychosocial problems in primary care: patient and provider perceptions. Soc Work Health Care [Internet]. 2009 Nov 20 [cited 2017 Oct 10];48(8):736–49. Available from: http://www.ncbi.nlm.nih.gov/pubmed/20182986.
46. Schor EL. Rethinking well-child care. Pediatrics. 2004;114(1):210 LP–216.
47. Thackeray J, Stelzner S, Downs SM, Miller C. Screening for intimate partner violence. J Interpers Violence [Internet]. 2007 Jun 2 [cited 2017 Oct 10];22(6):659–70. Available from: http://www.ncbi.nlm.nih.gov/pubmed/17515428.
48. Gottlieb L, Hessler D, Long D, Amaya A, Adler N. A randomized trial on screening for social determinants of health: the iScreen study. Pediatrics [Internet]. 2014 Dec 3 [cited 2017 Oct 10];134(6):e1611–8. Available from: http://www.ncbi.nlm.nih.gov/pubmed/25367545.

49. Mackenzie SLC, Kurth AE, Spielberg F, Severynen A, Malotte CK, St. Lawrence J, et al. Patient and staff perspectives on the use of a computer counseling tool for HIV and sexually transmitted infection risk reduction. J Adolesc Heal [Internet]. 2007 Jun [cited 2017 Oct 10];40(6):572.e9–572.e16. Available from: http://www.ncbi.nlm.nih.gov/pubmed/17531766.

50. Hussain N, Sprague S, Madden K, Hussain FN, Pindiprolu B, Bhandari M. A comparison of the types of screening tool administration methods used for the detection of intimate partner violence. Trauma, Violence, Abus [Internet]. 2015 Jan 15 [cited 2017 Oct 10];16(1):60–9. Available from: http://journals.sagepub.com/doi/10.1177/1524838013515759.

51. Connell CL, Lofton KL, Yadrick K, Rehner TA. Children's experiences of food insecurity can assist in understanding its effect on their well-being. J Nutr [Internet]. 2005 Jul [cited 2017 Sep 26];135(7):1683–90. Available from: http://www.ncbi.nlm.nih.gov/pubmed/15987850.

52. Fram MS, Frongillo EA, Jones SJ, Williams RC, Burke MP, DeLoach KP, et al. Children are aware of food insecurity and take responsibility for managing food resources. J Nutr [Internet]. 2011 Jun 1 [cited 2017 Sep 26];141(6):1114–9. Available from: http://www.ncbi.nlm.nih.gov/pubmed/21525257.

53. Bradley KA, Lapham GT, Hawkins EJ, Achtmeyer CE, Williams EC, Thomas RM, et al. Quality concerns with routine alcohol screening in VA clinical settings. J Gen Intern Med [Internet]. 2011 Mar [cited 2017 Oct 10];26(3):299–306. Available from: http://www.ncbi.nlm.nih.gov/pubmed/20859699.

54. Williams EC, Achtmeyer CE, Thomas RM, Grossbard JR, Lapham GT, Chavez LJ, et al. Factors underlying quality problems with alcohol screening prompted by a clinical reminder in primary care: a multi-site qualitative study. J Gen Intern Med [Internet]. 2015 Aug [cited 2017 Oct 10];30(8):1125–32. Available from: http://www.ncbi.nlm.nih.gov/pubmed/25731916.

55. Henize AW, Beck AF, Klein MD, Adams M, Kahn RS. A road map to address the social determinants of health through community collaboration. Pediatrics [Internet]. 2015 Sep 1 [cited 2017 Oct 10];peds.2015-0549. Available from: http://pediatrics.aappublications.org/content/early/2015/09/15/peds.2015-0549.

56. Beck AF, Klein MD, Kahn RS. Identifying social risk via a clinical social history embedded in the electronic health record. Clin Pediatr (Phila) [Internet]. 2012 Oct 17 [cited 2017 Oct 10];51(10):972–7. Available from: http://www.ncbi.nlm.nih.gov/pubmed/22511197.

57. Bazemore AW, Cottrell EK, Gold R, Hughes LS, Phillips RL, Angier H, et al. "Community vital signs": incorporating geocoded social determinants into electronic records to promote patient and population health. J Am Med Informatics Assoc [Internet]. 2016 Mar [cited 2017 Dec 11];23(2):407–12. Available from: http://www.ncbi.nlm.nih.gov/pubmed/26174867.

58. Troseth MR. American academy of nursing endorses social behavioral determinants of health in electronic health records. Comput Inform Nurs [Internet]. 2017 Jul [cited 2017 Dec 11];35(7):329–30. Available from: http://insights.ovid.com/crossref?an=00024665-201707000-00002.

59. Reed S, Shell R, Kassis K, Tartaglia K, Wallihan R, Smith K, et al. Applying adult learning practices in medical education. Curr Probl Pediatr Adolesc Health Care [Internet]. 2014 Jul [cited 2017 Dec 11];44(6):170–81. Available from: http://linkinghub.elsevier.com/retrieve/pii/S1538544214000182.

60. Russell SS. An overview of adult-learning processes. Urol Nurs [Internet]. 2006 Oct [cited 2017 Dec 11];26(5):349–52, 370. Available from: http://www.ncbi.nlm.nih.gov/pubmed/17078322.

61. O'Toole JK, Solan LG, Burkhardt MC, Klein MD. Watch and learn: an innovative video trigger curriculum to increase resident screening for social determinants of health. Clin Pediatr (Phila) [Internet]. 2013 Apr 7 [cited 2017 Dec 11];52(4):344–50. Available from: http://journals.sagepub.com/doi/10.1177/0009922813475702.

62. Knowles MS, Holton EF, Swanson RA. THE ADULT LEARNER the definitive classic in adult education and human resource development. Elsevier; 2005. 1–378 p.

63. Community Pediatrics Training Initiatives [Internet]. [cited 2017 Oct 27]. Available from: https://www.aap.org/en-us/advocacy-and-policy/aap-health-initiatives/CPTI/Pages/default.aspx.

64. U.S. Child Poverty Curriculum [Internet]. [cited 2017 Oct 13]. Available from: https://www. aap.org/en-us/advocacy-and-policy/aap-health-initiatives/CPTI/Pages/U-S-Child-Poverty-Curriculum.aspx.
65. Chamberlain LJ, Hanson ER, Klass P, Schickedanz A, Nakhasi A, Barnes MM, et al. Childhood poverty and its effect on health and well-being: enhancing training for learners across the medical education continuum. Acad Pediatr [Internet]. 2016 Apr [cited 2017 Dec 11];16(3):S155–62. Available from: http://www.ncbi.nlm.nih.gov/pubmed/27044694.
66. Klein MD, Alcamo AM, Beck AF, O'Toole JK, McLinden D, Henize A, et al. Can a video curriculum on the social determinants of health affect residents' practice and families' perceptions of care? Acad Pediatr [Internet]. 2014 Mar [cited 2017 Dec 11];14(2):159–66. Available from: http://linkinghub.elsevier.com/retrieve/pii/S1876285913003161.
67. LNCO Advocacy training [Internet]. Oregon Health & Science University. Available from: http://www.ohsu.edu/xd/health/services/doernbecher/research-education/education/pediatric-residency-program/program/advocacy.cfm.
68. O'Brien MJ, Garland JM, Murphy KM, Shuman SJ, Whitaker RC, Larson SC. Training medical students in the social determinants of health: the Health Scholars Program at Puentes de Salud. Adv Med Educ Pract [Internet]. 2014 Sep [cited 2017 Dec 11];5:307–14. Available from: http://www.dovepress.com/training-medical-students-in-the-social-determinants-of-health-the-hea-peer-reviewed-article-AMEP.
69. Northrip KD, Bush HM, Li H-F, Marsh J, Chen C, Guagliardo MF. Pediatric residents' knowledge of the community. Acad Pediatr [Internet]. 2012 Jul [cited 2017 Dec 11];12(4):350–6. Available from: http://linkinghub.elsevier.com/retrieve/pii/S1876285912000691.
70. Real FJ, Beck AF, Spaulding JR, Sucharew H, Klein MD. Impact of a neighborhood-based curriculum on the helpfulness of pediatric residents' anticipatory guidance to impoverished families. Matern Child Health J [Internet]. 2016 Nov 1 [cited 2017 Dec 11];20(11):2261–7. Available from: http://link.springer.com/10.1007/s10995-016-2133-7.
71. Community Health and Advocacy Rotation | BCRP | Boston Children's Hospital [Internet]. [cited 2017 Oct 11]. Available from: http://www.childrenshospital.org/bcrp/program/benefiting-the-community/community-health-and-advocacy-rotation.
72. Lujan HL, DiCarlo SE. First-year medical students prefer multiple learning styles. Adv Physiol Educ. 2006;30(1):13–6.
73. VARK Questionnaire [Internet]. [cited 2017 Dec 22]. Available from: http://vark-learn.com/the-vark-questionnaire/.
74. Palis AG, Quiros PA. Adult learning principles and presentation pearls. Middle East Afr J Ophthalmol [Internet]. 2014 [cited 2017 Dec 11];21(2):114–22. Available from: http://www. meajo.org/text.asp?2014/21/2/114/129748.
75. Real FJ, Michelson CD, Beck AF, Klein MD. Location, location, location: teaching about neighborhoods in pediatrics. Acad Pediatr [Internet]. 2017 Apr [cited 2017 Dec 11];17(3):228–32. Available from: http://www.ncbi.nlm.nih.gov/pubmed/27988207.
76. Blumberg SJ, Bialostosky K, Hamilton WL, Briefel RR. The effectiveness of a short form of the Household Food Security Scale. Am J Public Health [Internet]. 1999 Aug [cited 2017 Oct 8];89(8):1231–4. Available from: http://www.ncbi.nlm.nih.gov/pubmed/10432912.
77. Blumberg J Bialostosky K Hamilton W Briefel R. U.S. household food security survey module: six-item short form economic research service, USDA September 2012. Am J Public Health [Internet]. 1999;89:1231–4. Available from: https://www.ers.usda.gov/media/8282/short2012.pdf.
78. Billioux A. Standardized screening for health-related social needs in clinical settings the accountable health communities screening tool. 2017 [cited 2017 Oct 10]; Available from: https://nam.edu/wp-content/uploads/2017/05/Standardized-Screening-for-Health-Related-Social-Needs-in-Clinical-Settings.pdf.
79. Urke HB, Cao ZR, Egeland GM. Validity of a single item food security questionnaire in Arctic Canada. Pediatrics [Internet]. 2014 Jun 1 [cited 2017 Dec 11];133(6):e1616–23. Available from: http://www.ncbi.nlm.nih.gov/pubmed/24864166.

80. Nord M, Hopwood H. Recent advances provide improved tools for measuring children's food security. J Nutr [Internet]. 2007 Mar;137(3):533–6. Available from: http://proxygw.wrlc.org/login?url=http://search.ebscohost.com/login.aspx?direct=true&db=mdc&AN=17311935&site=eds-live&scope=site&authtype=ip,uid&custid=s8987071.

81. Kenyon C, Sandel M, Silverstein M, Shakir A, Zuckerman B. Revisiting the social history for child health. Pediatrics [Internet]. 2007 Sep 1 [cited 2017 Dec 11];120(3):e734–8. Available from: http://www.ncbi.nlm.nih.gov/pubmed/17766513.

82. Riddell J, Jhun P, Fung C-C, Comes J, Sawtelle S, Tabatabai R, et al. Does the flipped classroom improve learning in graduate medical education? J Grad Med Educ [Internet]. 2017 Aug [cited 2017 Dec 11];9(4):491–6. Available from: http://www.jgme.org/doi/10.4300/JGME-D-16-00817.1.

83. Community Pediatrics CO. Poverty and child health in the United States. Pediatrics [Internet]. 2016 Apr 1 [cited 2017 Dec 11];137(4):e20160339–e20160339. Available from: http://www.ncbi.nlm.nih.gov/pubmed/26962238.

84. Klein MD, Kahn RS, Baker RC, Fink EE, Parrish DS, White DC. Training in social determinants of health in primary care: does it change resident behavior? Acad Pediatr [Internet]. 2011;11(5):387–93. Available from: https://doi.org/10.1016/j.acap.2011.04.004

85. Klein M, Vaughn LM. Teaching social determinants of child health in a pediatric advocacy rotation: small intervention, big impact. Med Teach. 2010;32(9):754–9.

Chapter 3
Scope of Interventions to Address Food Insecurity

Janine S. Bruce, Deepak Palakshappa, and Hans B. Kersten

Abbreviations

AAP	American Academy of Pediatrics
ACGME	Accreditation Council for Graduate Medical Education
AMA	American Medical Association
CHW	Community health worker
EHR	Electronic health record
FI	Food Insecurity
FPL	Federal poverty level
SDH	Social Determinants of Health
SFSP	Summer Food Service Program
SNAP	Supplemental Nutrition Assistance Program
TANF	Temporary Assistance for Needy Families
WCC	Well-child check
WIC	Special Supplemental Nutrition Program for Women, Infants, and Children

J. S. Bruce
Stanford University School of Medicine, Stanford, CA, USA
e-mail: jsbruce@stanford.edu

D. Palakshappa
Wake Forest School of Medicine, Winston-Salem, NC, USA

H. B. Kersten (✉)
St. Christopher's Hospital for Children, Drexel University College of Medicine, Philadelphia, PA, USA
e-mail: hk39@drexel.edu

© The Author(s) 2018
H. B. Kersten et al. (eds.), *Identifying and Addressing Childhood Food Insecurity in Healthcare and Community Settings*, SpringerBriefs in Public Health, https://doi.org/10.1007/978-3-319-76048-3_3

Aim

1. Characterize three levels of intervention (individual, community, and policy) that give providers unique opportunities to reduce FI for their patients and families.

Case Study

A young mom, Sandra, brings her 6-month old daughter into the pediatric primary care center for a well-child check (WCC). Dad, Mateo, works as a day laborer and mom stays at home. She has brought her other two young sons (age 2 and 6) with her to the visit. Mom seems happy but tired. The children climb on the examination table as you come in; they excitedly look at the books you gave them during the visit. As part of your discussion during the visit, you turn to the social risk questionnaire completed as part of the WCC. You explain to mom why you ask about things like housing, support systems, and public benefits; you highlight why such factors are so important to the health of her children. As you review the 14-item questionnaire, you find that it is positive for food insecurity (FI). This leads you to ask some additional questions. You inquire about the family's financial situation. Mom says that dad does not make enough to feed the family; he is in and out of work. Dad is undocumented, so they only receive Supplemental Nutrition Assistance Program (SNAP) benefits for mom and the children. Additionally, mom says she stopped getting Special Supplemental Nutrition Program for Women, Infants, and Children (WIC) benefits since she finds it difficult to get to that office so frequently. In the past, they have considered dis-enrolling completely from programs like SNAP and WIC due to immigration fears in the community. Moreover, they do not seem to know about or access local community resources.

You contemplate these responses. You, and your colleagues at the primary care center, have only recently started screening for social risks like FI. You have learned about some key public programs and local agencies that can help families with FI and have compiled information to help families learn more about these programs. Still, you recognize key limitations: the WIC office can be difficult for some families to access. Also, although SNAP and WIC are evidence-based and effective programs for low-income families, they are susceptible to budgetary cuts often considered by policymakers. You make a note to yourself to learn of other ways to advocate for families like this one.

Rationale for Immediate Response

Healthcare providers are uniquely situated to screen for and address social determinants of health (SDH) [1, 2]. This potential role was recognized by a "rebel" of a pediatrician in the nineteenth Century named Abraham Jacobi who advocated for providing care for children in a holistic way [3]. Such care often requires identifying and addressing social alongside medical factors. A starting point is screening, which has been outlined in previous chapters. Screening must be recognized as just a start, however, and many providers would have been hard pressed to help families screening positive for a risk like FI just a few years ago. Often, we did not ask the question; when we did, we rarely knew how to respond.

Fortunately, we now have a better understanding of the relevance of social determinants on health outcomes. In parallel, we have a better sense of how we can more effectively provide targeted resources to our at-risk patients and families, linking those families to clinic- or community-based supports. Screening without such action would not only be "ineffective," it may also considered "unethical" by some [4].

Many healthcare providers are currently screening for and addressing SDH in their practice, but studies show few do so routinely [5, 6]. This is due, in part, to a lack of time or knowledge of how to respond to identified SDH-related risks. However, early research demonstrates that interventions can positively affect family circumstances and improve child health [6]. In order to effectively address risks like FI, healthcare providers need the right tools and skills [2]. They can support families in different ways: (1) as individuals practicing in clinical settings; (2) as partners in the community; and (3) through policy-level advocacy (Table 3.1) [7]. In this chapter, we will move from screening toward action, highlighting these three tiers of intervention that give healthcare providers unique opportunities to reduce FI for their patients and families.

In-Clinic Provider-Based Approach (Tier 1)

FI is a complex, multi-factorial social problem that has no single solution. Individual healthcare providers or clinicians seeing patients in healthcare settings, are uniquely situated to identify and address FI. Indeed, these providers (e.g., physicians, nurses, social workers) are well-positioned to screen for FI, and to link families to a diverse array of clinic- and community-based resources. Below, we outline key reflections as provider-directed interventions in clinical settings are considered (Tier 1). After discussion of the positive screen, interventions could range from giving families paper or electronic resource listings, providing food or a prescription for a box of food, connecting with on-site staff (e.g., social worker, legal advocate, or community health worker [CHW]), and referring families to community-based programs. Some clinics may even have on-site food pantries. Clearly, these interventions will carry different challenges and opportunities since they vary significantly in scope. Not all of these approaches may be needed, but each provider or clinical setting might develop or adapt tools and initiatives to effectively meet the needs of their patient panels.

Table 3.1 Multi-Tiered approach to addressing food insecurity

	Actions and solutions	Program leads	Trackable outcomes

Tier 1. In-clinic provider-based approach	• Resource list
	  • Create on own
	  • Use list from community partner
	• Encourage family to enroll in core public benefits like SNAP and WIC
	• Refer for emergency food box
	• Write prescription for box of fresh food
	• Write prescription for farm stand for $10 off purchase of produce
	• Consult social worker or office staff to help facilitate efforts
		• Healthcare providers
		• Clinical office staff
			• Number of resource lists distributed
			• Number of families enrolled in the fresh produce program
			  • of families accessing resources
			• Health, preventive service outcomes available from the EHR

Tier 2. Community-engaged approach	• Meet with key community agencies and organizations to enhance view of public and community-based resources • Engage in collaborative projects that support families' access and utilization of existing programs • Collaboratively develop new programs to fill identifiable gaps • Engage in longitudinal community-based participatory research to evaluate programs	• Healthcare providers • Social services agencies • Public benefits administrators • Food banks and pantries • Resource centers • Schools • Libraries	• Connections between agencies (number and strength) • Quality, accuracy of resource information for physicians to provide to families • Number of clinic-based referrals to partnered agencies • Number of individuals/families served or stories of personal experiences an barriers to utilizing food resources (qualitative data)
Tier 3. Advocacy-based approach	• Advocate for families during clinic visits • Work with local organizations or medical societies to advocate on a broader scale • Educate trainees about FI and other SDH	• Healthcare providers • Local, state and federal officials • Media	• Extent of deployment of curriculum that teaches residents about how to address FI in practice • Number of op-eds written • Number of meetings with elected officials • Policy changes

Now, let us consider the resources healthcare providers have in clinical settings, or supports to which they can connect their patients, to address positive FI screens in their clinical setting.

In-Clinic FI-Relevant Resources

One of the most important tools to help address FI is the electronic health record (EHR), a robust data collection and tracking tool now common to healthcare delivery sites. Many practices now incorporate their social risk screening into their EHR, putting such vital information directly in front of providers as they pursue their care. At a practice level, tracking FI through EHRs can allow healthcare providers and administrators to assess trends in FI levels over time, informing provider- and clinic-level front-line practice changes and interventions. EHRs can also link families to resources [8, 9], but more evidence is needed to determine how such linkages can best occur and how they affect outcomes [10].

Another tool that should be readily available when discussing a positive FI screen is a list of community resources. This may be in the form of a paper handout or online links to resources. A resource list can include contact information for local food banks or pantries, local hunger organizations that often distribute emergency food, and enrollment information for important public benefit programs (e.g., SNAP, WIC, Temporary Assistance for Needy Families [TANF]). Researching and creating such a list can be incredibly informative when a provider begins screening for FI. However, it can be quite onerous to keep it updated. Fortunately, many local hunger organizations often have updated lists that can be adapted or used within clinical settings (Fig. 3.1). Such organizations are often very willing to partner with healthcare providers to develop tailored lists and resources for particular settings or geographic areas. These partnerships can ease the effort needed to keep an updated list on hand while also establishing relationships with potential community-based collaborators (see Tier 2 below).

Lastly, healthcare providers commonly prescribe medicines. Now, some innovative programs are using prescriptions as a way for providers to link families to needed resources or improve access to fresh fruit and vegetable programs [11–13]. Support for such a prescription could be supported by a collaborative community partner, facilitating a connection that may have otherwise been difficult; perhaps it could also include nutrition education and cooking demonstrations that would integrate community health resources into the healthcare setting. Moreover, the concept of prescribing food, using food as medicine, elevates the perceived importance of nutrition as a key component of health and well-being. Although more research is clearly needed, prescriptions for food have been shown to increase fruit and vegetable consumption, reduce FI, and improve the health of patients [11–17].

The EHR can be readily used to screen and track positive FI screens and may develop a program to use prescriptions to link families to fresh produce.

Save Money & Eat Healthier!

 Greater Philadelphia Coalition Against Hunger
215-430-0556
www.hungercoalition.org

 Call our Hotline 215-430-0556 for free, confidential service to:
- Check your eligibility for SNAP (food stamps) and apply by phone
- Get help with problems with your benefits
- Find pantries and other food programs in your area

 FOR FAMILIES WITH CHILDREN

WIC (Women, Infants and Children) Program: Helps pregnant women and mothers with children under age 5 with food, health screenings and nutritional information. 1-800-743-3300, www.northwic.org

Maternity Care Coalition: Provides baby formula and other services. 215-972-0700, http://momobile.org

Free Summer Meals for Kids (June-August): Free meals & snacks for kids 18 & under. No registration required. To find a site, call 1-855-252-MEAL (6325), text "FOOD" to 877877, or visit www.phillysummermeals.org

 FOR SENIORS or PEOPLE AT NUTRITIONAL RISK DUE TO ILLNESS

Philadelphia Corporation for the Aging: Provides meals at senior centers and delivers meals to eligible seniors. Gives out farmers' market vouchers at various locations. 215-765-9040, www.pcacares.org

Aid For Friends: Delivers free meals to isolated homebound individuals. 215-464-2224, www.aidforfriends.org

MANNA: Delivers meals to people at nutritional risk due to illness. Dietitians provide free nutritional counseling. A referral is required from a medical care provider. 215-496-2662 x5, www.mannapa.org

 FREE OR DISCOUNTED FOOD OR PRODUCE

SHARE Food Program: Get $50 in groceries for $20-30 plus 2 hours of community service. Accepts SNAP (food stamps) and farmers' market vouchers. 215-223-2220, www.sharefoodprogram.org

Jewish Relief Agency (JRA): Delivers a free box of kosher food once a month, regardless of religious affiliation. Recipients must live within JRA's service area in Philadelphia and surrounding counties. 610-660-0190, www.jewishrelief.org

Fresh for All: Philabundance (www.philabundance.org) offers free produce year-round, weather permitting. No ID or registration is required, but you must bring your own bag, box or cart. Days and locations include:
- *Thursday 10:30-11:30am, Houseman Recreation Center, Summerdale & Godfrey Avenues, Northeast Philly*
- *Friday 1:30-2:30pm, at the lot under the I-95 overpass at Front and Tasker Streets, South Philly*

GREATER PHILADELPHIA COALITION AGAINST HUNGER | 215-430-0556 | WWW.HUNGERCOALITION.ORG

Fig. 3.1 An example of a healthy food resource list from the Greater Philadelphia Coalition Against Hunger

However, healthcare providers should have an understanding of public benefit programs and key community food programs. They may also consider engagement with additional clinic personnel that could help families with positive FI screens.

Key Public Benefit Programs

Discussion about addressing FI in the office should begin with widely available programs that have been shown to reduce FI in families. SNAP, a public benefit for low-income families, provides more nutritional assistance than any other program [18]. More than a quarter of U.S. families currently participate in SNAP; >50% participate in SNAP at some time in their life. Enrollment in SNAP is also an evidence-based tool that has many benefits (Table 3.2). Families qualify if their gross income is <130% of the federal poverty level (FPL). SNAP provides a modest benefit ($1.35 per person per meal), but it lifts millions of children out of poverty each year. This supplement has been shown to improve child health and school performance while also stimulating the local economy [9, 18]. SNAP is federally funded and is available in every state. Given its proven effectiveness and relevance to food insecure households, we encourage healthcare providers and clinics to familiarize themselves with SNAP's eligibility requirements, being aware that some will not qualify due to income or immigration restrictions. Also, given its supplemental nature, many who receive SNAP benefits will still be food insecure. Thus, familiarity with other programs is important.

Another evidence-based benefit is WIC, a state-run program that serves low-income pregnant women and children less than 5 years old (Table 3.2). Families with household incomes ≤185% of the FPL qualify. WIC provides infant formula, milk, and fresh produce to families. The program has been shown to encourage healthier eating, improve early childhood development and long-term academic achievement, and reduce household FI [9]. Connecting potentially-eligible families to SNAP and WIC should be a priority to pediatric healthcare providers and their teams.

Of course, WIC does not cover those children who have reached school age. Fortunately, additional public programs commence at this stage, including the school meals, afterschool snack, and summer food programs (Table 3.2). Households with incomes below <185% FPL can receive reduced price school meals and those <130% FPL can receive free meals. These programs have been shown to reduce FI, obesity and poor health. Participation may be limited since students have to show their families' income, but many districts have universal meals to increase participation and reduce costs [9, 18].

Despite the availability and importance of public programs like SNAP, WIC, and the school-based programs, families often face multiple barriers to participation. Generally, barriers include not meeting eligibility criteria and not having sufficient information about how to apply or participate (e.g., complicated enrollment, limited access to food even with the benefit). Public agencies and community-based organi-

Table 3.2 Description of key state and national programs to address food insecurity

Program	Overview	Eligibility	Indication	Contact
Supplemental nutrition assistance program (SNAP)	• Entitlement program, previously known as food stamps, that provides nutrition assistance to families and individuals • Largest nutrition assistance program • Participants receive a monthly benefits, loaded on an electronic benefit transfer card, to purchase food	• Variable by state, but generally a gross income <130% of the federal poverty level • Asset test may apply in some states (e.g., how much an individual has in resources, if they own a car)	Long-term	https://www.fns.usda.gov/snap/state-informationhotline-numbers
Special supplemental nutrition program for women, infants, and children (WIC)	• Provides federal grants to states for supplemental foods, nutrition education, and referrals to healthcare and social services • Families receive food packages each month	• Women if they are pregnant, postpartum, or breastfeeding • Infants are eligible through 1 year old • Children are eligible through 5 years old • Household income • ≤185% of the FPL • Automatically eligible if receive Medicaid, SNAP, or TANF	Long-term	https://www.fns.usda.gov/wic/wic-contacts
Temporary assistance for needy families (TANF)	• Block grant program that provides money for states to fund work and family support programs • Provides assistance for families so that children can be cared for at home and promote job preparation	• Varies by state • Often have specific work and job preparation provisions	Long-term	https://www.acf.hhs.gov/ofa/programs/tanf

Program	Description	Timeframe	Resources
National School Lunch and breakfast program	• Federal funding is provided to schools to offer free or reduced price meals to children from low or moderate income families • 32 million children a year receive free or reduced price lunch • 13 million children a year receive free or reduced price breakfast	• Children and adolescents kindergarten through 12th grade • Households <185% FPL receive reduce price; households <130% FPL receive free meals • Community eligibility provision allows schools in areas of high poverty to offer free breakfast and lunch to all students	Immediate and long-term	www.frac.org/aaptoolkit https://www.fns.usda.gov/nslp/national-school-lunch-program-nslp
Child and adult care food program	• Federal assistance to states to provide nutrition foods to child and adult care institutions • Funds free meals and snacks for children in child care centers, family child care homes, and head start or early head start programs	• Children who attend eligible child care centers and homes	Immediate and long term	www.frac.org/aaptoolkit https://www.fns.usda.gov/cacfp/child-and-adult-care-food-program
Summer food service program	• Federal assistance to approved community sites to offer free meals and snacks during the summer • Sites offer educational, enrichment, physical and recreational activities • Summer meal sites must be located in a low-income area or serve a majority of children who qualify for free or reduced price school meals	• Children 18 years of age and younger can receive free meals and snacks at approved community sites	Short-term	https://www.fns.usda.gov/sfsp/summer-food-service-program www.frac.org/aaptoolkit

zations are critical extenders that can, at times, overcome these barriers, supporting outreach and enrollment [11]. We contend that healthcare providers and their teams can be similar extenders, connectors to these other organizations in ways that support families as they use or enroll in these critical benefit programs or other community-based food agencies and programs.

Community Food Programs

Healthcare providers (and clinics) can also connect with local community-based organizations and food programs to support their patients and families. Food banks and pantries can provide additional information or an emergency food supply to their patients. Different sites often have different eligibility criteria and hours, so the Feeding America site is a great place to start: the zip code where the family lives can be entered to see what food banks are in the area [19]. The local food bank may then have lists and contact information for the food pantries it serves within a region, a list that is easily shared with families. Other community resources may be available online or via the phone. Many cities have a means through which general inquiries can be made for social needs. The 211 line is a universal number for community services and referrals. This service is more robust in some places when compared to another, but it may be a reasonable place to start with a social needs question. They may even have answers about where families could get food in an emergency. Similarly, in many locations, calling 311 directly connects citizens with the government who may be able to help them find food or other resources they need.

Resources such as these, ranging from food banks and pantries to community extenders, are present across the country. For example, Greater Philadelphia's Coalition Against Hunger provides an extended list of area food pantries [20]. Philabundance is a Philadelphia-based food bank and social service organization that distributes food, raises awareness, and advocates for hunger issues [21]. Philadelphia's SHARE Food Program distributes boxes of fresh produce for minimal cost [22]. A final example, is the "cap4kids" website which lists hundreds of resources for healthcare providers and families to access [23]. Pages can be printed for FI or many other SDH that the pediatric provider encounters. This site, which started in Philadelphia, is now available for many sites across the country (http://cap4kids.org).

Information on public benefits and community-based programs may all find their way to the resource list that was discussed above. Of course, just giving such a list to a family may be insufficient. Such an approach relies on families to gather and process information, and then seek out connections to named resources. For some, this step can be a stumbling block given barriers associated with finding necessary time and transportation. Others may find that eligibility, complex enrollment processes, or immigration fears are additional barriers that may be, or seem, insurmountable [24–28].

Any effort to address FI requires collaborative, multi-faceted, innovative strategies that can support diverse, often hard-to-reach populations. The use of additional types of providers in the clinical setting could help the clinic extend their reach. A discussion of such additional personnel follows.

Additional Clinic Personnel

There are many types of providers who can help healthcare providers care for families confronting FI. A team approach is becoming the standard way to approach FI and other SDH, but there are many types of teams which can vary with available personnel and expertise [9]. Some clinics may be "resource-rich," with a multi-disciplinary team capable of a range of potential actions. Others may be more "resource-limited," forced to consider those other connectors that may exist outside the clinical walls.

That said, social workers have long been important members of clinical teams. They often have tremendous knowledge of public benefit programs and community-based organizations. They can also augment the ability of healthcare providers by spending more time with families in the office and pursuing more in-depth risk screening [9, 29]. Some have used an alternative, "help desk" model. This model, most commonly associated with Health Leads™, involves non-professionals (e.g., college students) working with families with unmet social needs. Families are referred to the help desk where the volunteer helps actively connect families to community resources. This approach has been shown to improve health outcomes when patients are linked to basic resources [2, 9]. Still, social workers and on-site volunteers may not always be able to follow up with families after they leave the clinical setting. Some have access to CHWs, those who can bridge the gap between the healthcare provider's office and the families' home to assist with their needs. They may meet the family in the office and go into the home to help connect families with services. This more intensive approach has been shown to improve the social needs and the reported health status of families [6, 30]. Some insurance payers have begun to support the utilization of CHWs to address the social needs of the highest healthcare utilizers.

Many low-income families also have legal needs that can significantly affect their families' health and well-being [31]. An example of relevance to FI is public benefit denial or delay. Certain children (and households) may have been unfairly, or illegally, denied SNAP despite applying in the appropriate manner. This represents a FI-related legal need, one that many low-income families will find themselves unable to counter. Medical-legal partnerships are an emerging strategy that bridges legal advocates with clinical practices. This model enables healthcare and legal professionals to collaboratively address SDH in innovative ways to positively affect clinical systems and improve the care of these families [9, 31].

Although many models have shown great promise, addressing FI and other SDH is relatively new for providers, clinics, and healthcare systems. The best and most effective methods to help families has yet to be determined. It will likely take providers connecting families in multiple different ways to help families with so many different abilities and challenges [2, 11]. We have seen in Tier 1 how healthcare providers can get started within their setting. Now we will turn to considerations of how those action steps can bridge to the community to address FI through longitudinal collaborations.

Community-Engaged Approach (Tier 2)

Given the complexity of FI, multiple approaches are needed to provide children and families with the necessary resources and support to address their nutritional needs. The healthcare provider-based approaches (*Tier 1*) described above are excellent at offering immediate support to families, helping them connect to public and community-based programs, and to other local resources (Table 3.1). That said, a family's ability to adequately access and utilize resources may be fraught with interpersonal, systems, and eligibility barriers. Community agencies and organizations provide families with numerous levels of support ranging from providing referral information, to direct support for services including assistance with program enrollment (i.e., connections to and/or help filling out SNAP or WIC applications), nutrition education, food distribution, and hot meals. Thus, healthcare providers have the opportunity to step outside of the clinic walls, to be a key partner at the community level, actively engaging with a host of different agencies and organizations to collectively address FI within communities (*Tier 2*).

Leaders in pediatrics view this deeper engagement as beneficial for delivering effective community training to learners, such as residents and medical students, and on collaboratively reducing community-level health risks [32]. Healthcare providers interested in community-engaged approaches often develop and sustain authentic long-term community partnerships with agencies and organizations that are similarly focused on addressing issues of FI. At this level of engagement, collaborative work around shared priority areas should include the presence of shared values, mutually identified strategies, and partnerships that embody shared respect, inclusiveness, equal power sharing, and the possibility of mutual benefit [33].

Together, healthcare providers and community partners form community-academic partnerships that leverage the unique skills and expertise of various participants to advance a common goal. Partnerships go beyond simple referrals, focusing more on how a multi-disciplinary team can work together to develop and implement innovative collaborative efforts that meet community-identified needs. Working together, aligned partners can leverage their unique and complementary skills, expertise, and resources to synergistically address FI. The strategies and actions that follow have the potential to better serve populations while simultaneously improving health in equitable ways [34, 35]. With this in mind, we outline, below, specific strategies and opportunities that could be used to develop and sustain long-term community collaborative partnerships.

- *Ask and Listen:* One of the first steps in developing community partnerships is meeting with community partner organizations to ask and listen. First, ask about the needs of their target population and community partner priority areas, and then listen without interjecting. Healthcare providers can ask partners what needs families face and what priority strategies these organizations are undertaking to meet these needs. This requires healthcare partners to humbly listen as equal partners, rather than experts with all of the answers. This act of "listening" demonstrates to community partners that they are viewed as experts given their strong connection to the individuals and populations they serve.
- *Identify Unique Skills Healthcare Providers can Leverage*: Healthcare providers can also identify unique skills, expertise, and leveraged resources they can bring to the partnership. Depending on the community-identified need, healthcare providers can help communities identify and articulate the needs of the target population by conducting formal or informal needs assessments. Additionally, they can help community members or agencies rigorously evaluate program outputs and outcomes, an area often neglected when time or expertise is limited. Given their access to highly vulnerable populations, healthcare providers are also uniquely positioned to bear witness to the struggles and challenges of the children and families they serve. They can share stories with collaborative partners and policymakers that illustrate the real effects of FI on children and families.
- *Engage in Long-term Community Collaborations*: Healthcare providers have the opportunity to engage in long-term community collaboration. They can work alongside community partners to identify community needs, shared priorities, and potentially-useful strategies and interventions. For example, they can conduct or support needs assessments and the development of strategic plans, facilitate linkages to other aligned organizations, and support applications for collaborative funding. Once partnerships are formed, community partners can regularly reach out to healthcare providers for assistance on collaborative initiatives, viewing providers as a critical partner in the fight to eliminate local FI. The capacity to develop and sustain long-term partnerships has the potential to amplify both the mutual benefit to collaborative partners and the overall impact of collaborative efforts (Table 3.3).
- *Strive for Collective Impact:* Collective impact is based on the belief that large-scale social change requires sustained, broad coordination and leadership across multiple sectors (i.e., public or governmental agencies, for-profit and not-for-profit organizations, schools, universities, community members) united by a common mission [36]. Leaders must share a willingness to abandon individual goals and engage in collective agenda setting to establish shared priorities for meeting the needs of the community. The collective impact model also recognizes the contributions of each individual and organization, applying collaborative and evidence-based decision-making. Key to facilitating collective impact includes creation of a centralized infrastructure and staff, continuous communication, a structured process for accomplishing a shared agenda, shared measures and outcomes, and alignment of financial and other resources. Collective impact,

Table 3.3 Spectrum of long-term community collaborations

Intervention	Objectives	Physician engagement
Clinic-based WIC program	• Establish clinic-based WIC office	• Assess patient needs for co-located WIC services • Bring together WIC and clinic administrators to discuss common goals and collaborative opportunity
Clinic-based food pantry	• Establish a clinic-based food pantry or distribution program	• Conduct needs assessment among patients for a co-located food pantry • Partner with food bank, hospital food vendor, or grocery store to distribute or sell fresh fruits and vegetables
Clinic-based farmers market	• Establish a local farmers market on clinic property	• Conduct needs assessment among patients for a co-located farmers market • Bring together farmers market representatives, local food bank and clinic administrators to discuss collaborative opportunity • Develop a subsidized voucher program for patients utilizing farmers market • Partner to assess quantitative and qualitative outputs and outcomes
Clinic or hospital-based meal programs	• Serve free meals to low-income children and parents at clinics or hospitals	• Conduct needs assessment of clinic and/or hospital food insecurity among patients and families • Partner with community agency (e.g., food bank, meal program sponsor) or hospital food vendor to serve free meals to low-income children using public funding mechanism • Identify opportunities to leverage private funding for meals for low-income parents
Food prescription	• Develop food prescriptions for distribution at clinic	• Collaborate with food banks and other key partners create food prescription pad (handout) with pertinent food resource and contact information • Clearly indicate that the prescription is physician endorsed
Food resource guide	• Develop a hyper-local food resource guide • Distribute guide at clinic and in the community	• Partner with local food bank, schools, community organizations, churches, etc. to support access to existing food resources (e.g., pantries, school backpack programs, summer or weekend meals) • Develop food resource guide to be distributed at clinic and widely throughout community
Physician advocacy	• Participate in local FI collaboratives and task forces	• Serve as physician members of local community and school-based collaboratives and task forces aimed at addressing FI • Provide leadership in developing such collaboratives when none exist by serving as a convener • Leverage unique access to vulnerable populations and bear witness to the FI needs of patients and families
Community-based participatory research(33, 35)	• Engage in collaborative research that equitably involves partners in all phases of the research	• Identify opportunities to strengthen collaborative work by engaging in community-based, rigorous research to demonstrate impact • Leverage access to academic resources, while promoting a mutual exchange of expertise and resources among partners • Promote shared and equitable decision-making, ownership of the research process, funding, and dissemination of findings • Support community efforts to "take action" based on the research findings

when achieved, not only results in long-term partnerships but also the ability to assess improvements across shared indicators of success [36, 37]. Healthcare providers are well versed in coordinating care across multiple clinical disciplines. They can bring this perspective to their community-engaged work, amplifying the potential for larger sustained collective impact.

Example Model of Collaboration

There are times when such partnerships can originate within the clinical setting (see Chap. 4 for more information). What follows, however, is a case study of a collaborative community-based model for addressing childhood FI that was built by multiple organizations uniting for action within a community. This example demonstrates how a diverse group of individuals and organizations came together to address a shared priority issue, bringing their complementary expertise together while working toward a common vision.

Problem

At the height of the recession in 2012, a pediatrician working at a Bay Area Federally Qualified Health Center was seeing an increasing number of hungry families. She reported that one breastfeeding mother, in tears, recounted how she would regularly forgo meals so that her other children have enough to eat. Feeling helpless, the pediatrician and her colleagues reached out to the local school district to better understand the problem and identify possible opportunities to collaborate and intervene. Not surprisingly, the school's Director of Student Services was similarly worried about growing rates of FI among their children and families. The Director cited that overwhelmed teachers knew exactly which students were hungry in their class.

When asked what the local clinic and children's hospital could do to support local children and families, the Director asked for help feeding children during the summer. School administrators were extremely worried that students who relied on free and reduced-priced meals throughout the school year would experience heightened FI during the summer. Administrators recognized that many families experience added financial strain during summer months when child care and food costs often increase.

Partnership Development

In the first year of the resulting program, the primary partner organizations were the school district, food vendor, and a group of pediatricians from neighboring children's hospital. In subsequent years, the collaborative grew to comprise other key partners including a food bank, libraries, after-school programs, and other community agencies like the YMCA. The growing collaborative had the shared goal of reducing childhood FI in low-income, underserved communities. The collaborative specifically aimed to develop and implement innovative community-based approaches to increase child participation in the Summer Food Service Program (SFSP).

Move Toward Collaborative Action

A public-private partnership was developed to design and implement summer meal programs that utilized SFSP funding. All partners agreed that FI is a family issue, one that required a solution that served both children and adults. Since the first collaborative meal program was implemented in 2012, multiple models for the program have been tested.

1. School-based Meals: The first summer meal program was implemented in a local school district where >90% of children were eligible for free and reduced-priced meals. The program was held at a school that already housed a summer school program. The school was designated as an "open meal site," which allowed for reimbursement for all participating child meals given that the site operated in a low-income area where at least half of the children come from families with incomes ≤185% of the FPL.
2. Lunch at the Library: During the second summer, a local library began serving summer meals to children and adults, as they too were seeing increasing FI among library patrons. The library-based program targeted families utilizing library resources and/or participating in library-sponsored programs (e.g., reading time, summer camps for children, classes for adults). The program reached families not already affiliated or comfortable using school-based resources. It was later expanded to include meals during the winter holiday break and year-round meals at selected sites.
3. After School & Summer Camps: Several trusted partners provided summer meals through afterschool and summer camps run by the YMCA, Boys and Girls Clubs, and City Parks and Recreation programs. Providing summer meals through existing youth-oriented enrichment programs promoted food security while also preventing summer learning loss.
4. Mobile Meals: Targeting the hardest to reach families has continued to be an issue important to the collaborative. A mobile meal program that goes to local parks and popular community sites is a new model for reaching children and families where they are mostly likely to congregate during the summer months.
5. Community Food Resources: The collaborative worked together to develop food resource guides and outreach materials to better link families to existing public and community-based programs like public benefits and existing food pantries. These resources and materials were distributed at the aforementioned summer meals sites, schools, clinics, and other trusted community organizations.

Funding

One of the biggest barriers to leveraging SFSP funding for child meals during the summer has been the stringent and arduous federal reporting requirements. In this collaborative, the YMCA took the lead role in providing federal sponsorship for many of the participating program sites. Over the years, they have also trained many organizations to become their own federal sponsors, creating much needed capacity and sustainability. Funding for adult meals was provided through outside funding from the local food bank, children's hospital, and broader academic medical center.

Collective Impact

From the inception of the SFSP, the number of meals provided to children and adults increased from 13,000 in year one (school-based only), to >200,000 in year six (schools, libraries, after-school, summer camps, mobile sites). The number of collaborative partners has also expanded from three organizations to more than 15. The provision of adult meals at select sites has been maintained with ongoing support from the local food bank. Positive acknowledgment by local public officials has brought additional support and publicity for the program.

Lessons Learned

Key to the success of the collaborative was the shared goal of eliminating childhood FI. This goal, along with strong leadership, helped to unite partners from multiple sectors and organizations. Together, the partners learned how important it is to: (1) Identify trusted organizations and sites where families feel most comfortable; (2) Recognize and leverage unique skills and expertise among all collaborative partners; (3) Prioritize strong communication; and (4) Support transparent data sharing and dissemination. Partners also confirmed barriers faced by many program clients while also identifying new local, regional, and national challenges many faced. Such challenges highlight the need for advocacy, the need for healthcare providers (and partners) to speak out for children and families.

Advocacy-Based Approach (Tier 3)

Along with addressing families' needs at the provider and community levels, healthcare providers can also help their patients and families address FI through advocacy. Numerous national organizations, including the American Medical Association (AMA), the American Academy of Pediatrics (AAP), and the Accreditation Council for Graduate Medical Education (ACGME), consider advocacy to be a part of clinician's professional responsibilities [38–40]. The AAP defines advocacy as "the ongoing process of supporting or working towards a cause, an idea, or a policy." Clinicians have historically advocated at the federal level in support of nutrition assistance programs, such as SNAP, WIC, and the school-meals program [41]. Healthcare providers will need to continue to advocate across levels to maintain and expand such FI-relevant nutrition assistance programs (Table 3.2).

Healthcare providers are uniquely positioned to function as public advocates for health and well-being [38, 42]. The public trust in healthcare providers is high, and providers are viewed as a credible source of information. Given their social standing, clinicians often have increased access to policymakers, local or national leaders, and the broader citizenry. Because of their training and occupation, healthcare providers also have firsthand knowledge of the detrimental effects that FI and other SDH can have on patients' lives (see Chap. 1) [38, 43]. Providers can utilize this trust, access, and knowledge to advocate and support their patients by educating community leaders and policymakers about how risks like FI affect their patients' health. Healthcare providers can also use data to explain the impact of FI on children and families. For example, institutions who have implemented FI screening can describe the prevalence of FI in their patient populations to local leaders or the percentage of patients who are food insecure but ineligible for SNAP. It is critical for the success of child nutrition programs to maintain such a strong evidence base [41]. Local, state, and federal leaders and policymakers often want to know about both the personal impact of FI (i.e., qualitative patient stories) and the evidence on the effects of FI on health outcomes (i.e., quantitative data), which healthcare providers can provide.

Methods Healthcare Providers Can Use to Advocate

Although national organizations, medical societies, and clinicians recognize the importance of advocacy, there is no specific method for what it could or should entail [38, 42]. Healthcare providers are well acquainted with advocating for their individual patients. For example, taking extra steps to ensure that a patient is scheduled for a test or calling the pharmacy to ensure a parent receives a specific medication for their child are all tasks healthcare providers pursue nearly every day [44]. Advocacy to address FI likely requires more, or different, efforts than providing services for an individual patient or family. Indeed, it may require a broader perspective to address the root causes of the problems families face.

Although healthcare providers often positively endorse the idea of advocacy and civic engagement, there is limited data that healthcare providers engage in these activities. Potential reasons why there may be a gap between endorsing and engaging in clinician-advocacy include: time, social desirability (clinicians may say advocacy is important without deeply holding these views), fear of being in conflict with their institution, or concerns about how to effectively advocate [38, 42, 45, 46].

Advocacy may also be often considered narrowly, thought of as just lobbying or meeting with policymakers. In actuality, there are many forms of advocacy, and below, we discuss several methods healthcare providers can use to advocate to address the unmet food needs of their patients and families.

Educate Students and the Local Community

For clinics, hospitals, or healthcare systems with students and/or residents, educating the next generation of healthcare providers about FI and other SDH can be a key step in advocacy [9, 41]. Often, trainees do not have any prior training or knowledge about FI or SDH. Formal training in community health is associated with increased trainee involvement in community practices in the future [47]. This can include involving trainees in providing on-site resources to address FI, quality improvement initiatives (discussed further in Chap. 4) to improve screening efforts, or curriculum-based community site visits [41, 48]. Information about formal curricula to educate trainees are already available [48–50]. Interested individuals and institutions, with or without trainees, could also work to educate the local community. This could include placing signage within a practice about the rates of FI and its effects on child health. It could mean discussing the local prevalence and impact of FI with community members and leaders.

Work with a Medical Society, Community Partner, or Hunger Task Force

Healthcare providers can also advocate for food insecure families through local, state, or national organizations. This can include an individual's medical society, such as the AAP. Providers or institutions can also work with community partners to collaboratively advocate and support policies to address FI. Many local organizations or governments also have "hunger" or "poverty" task forces that could be a way to effect change in the community [9, 38, 41]. Developing a strategic partnership with a local organization can be an effective approach to increase recognition of and enhance policies addressing FI, exemplified in many ways by the case description of the SFSP above.

Summarize Clinical or Health Information for a Lay Audience

Educating the community or a lay audience about the negative impact of FI on child health can also be pursued through media outlets. Community leaders and policymakers are often unfamiliar with scientific articles relevant to FI or other child health issues. Healthcare providers can summarize scientific data and, perhaps, augment those data with patient stories to illustrate the extent of the problem. This could include an op-ed or a letter to the editor in a local or national newspaper. Op-eds and letters to the editor are opinion pieces that express an author's views about a particular topic, and they can be a good way to summarize an issue for a lay audience. Another media type is a blog post. A blog is a type of online journal or diary that allows an author to express her or his thoughts about a particular topic. Many organizations (e.g., Feeding America) have their own blogs, and a clinician could discuss the medical implications of a particular policy or topic (Table 3.4). A healthcare provider could also start her or his own blog either as an individual or at their institution to advocate for practices and policies to reduce FI and support child nutrition.

Table 3.4 Example blog post about the Community Eligibility Provision and how a change could effect patients and families like those introduced in this chapter

Today, I saw a 6-month-old patient whose family is struggling with having enough food at home. Even with her father working and the government assistance the family receives, it is still not enough for her parents and two other siblings to have enough food to eat at home. One of her siblings receives free meals at school, and I recently became aware of a bill that came out the house education and workforce committee called *Improving Child Nutrition and Education Act of 2016* (H.R. 5003). The bill contains several provisions that could negatively affect children's health and nutrition. Several organizations, including the American Academy of Pediatrics, oppose the bill. of particular concern is the bill raises the eligibility threshold for the community eligibility provision, which `allows schools to provide free breakfast and lunch for all students in high poverty areas. Schools where more than 40% of students are eligible for the federal school meals program are able to qualify to have the entire student population receive free meals. The new bill would increase the threshold to 60% eliminating free meals for thousands of students and worsening the food security for many.

The U.S. Department of Agriculture defines food insecurity (FI) as the lack of access to enough food for an active, healthy life. FI affects 16 million children in the U.S. and has been associated with many negative consequences in children including anemia, parental report of poor health, psychosocial and behavioral problems and poor academic performance. The National School Meals program is one federal resource that has improved the food security of many children and families by providing free or low-cost meals for students. Students automatically qualify for the school meals program if their families receive the supplemental nutrition assistance program (SNAP or food stamps), the temporary assistance for needy families (TANF), or similar programs. the community eligibility provision was established by the healthy, hunger-free kids act in 2010 and allows schools in high poverty areas to offer free breakfast and lunch to all students, thus eliminating the stigmatizing school meal application and providing savings for schools in administrative costs.

Raising the income threshold for the community eligibility provision from 40% to 60% would prevent more than 7000 of the 18,000 schools currently participating in the program and more than 3 million children, in low-income communities, could lose their access to school meals. While the bill would likely not affect the poorest students, schools that serve lower income communities would likely still suffer – Importantly, FI and hunger are not only found in the poorest communities. The "working poor" are likely to lose their access to free school meals with the passage of H.R. 5003. I urge you to call or write your congressman and tell them not to support H.R. 5003. This bill will only make it harder for hungry children to get access to food.

Reaching Out to Policymakers or Congressional Representatives

Another method to advocate and support FI programs is to reach out to or meet with policymakers or representatives at the local, state, or federal levels. Prior knowledge about which agency, branch, or level of government is responsible for appropriations or authorization of a particular FI-relevant program can help identify who to target. Outreach could include letters to a policy or decision maker. Often "click-based" campaigns are available, which will electronically submit letters to congressional leaders about a certain topic. Another method of outreach could be calling or meeting with an elected representative or staffer. Some tips to remember when talking to a representative, is to have a clear ask (such as "I want the senator to support X bill which will increase funding for Y benefits."). Use data to support why you think it is important (such as "15% of my patients are food insecure and this directly affects children's health and parents' ability to purchase medications."), and also include specific stories about how FI affects children and families (such as "I'm here because my 6-year old patient's family doesn't have enough food at home. Because of this lack of food, he keeps coming to my office with stomach pains and missing school."). Congressional representatives often trust the opinions of medical professionals, and healthcare providers can utilize their expertise and experiences to support programs to address FI.

Case Solutions

Tier 1. Clinic-Based Approach

Helping families get linked to necessary resources before they leave the clinical setting can be a crucial addition to care. There are a number of ways providers can help Sandra and her family right after FI is identified. The scope will depend on the resources available to providers in their practice. In the case introduced at the start of this chapter, the provider handed Sandra a resource list with information on places to get food urgently (Fig. 3.1). The handout also included criteria outlining whether her child would qualify for WIC along with contact information for the local WIC office. In addition to the resource list, the provider also printed a digital prescription (FreshRX) for a local Farm to Families program directly from the clinic's EHR. The provider explained that the program provides weekly boxes of fresh produce from local farms which can be purchased using SNAP benefits. The prescription also served as a $10 coupon for a Farm Stand set up at the weekly distribution site for produce. Finally, Sandra was linked to the on-site social worker for help with the WIC application, and confirmation that the family was receiving the proper amount of SNAP benefits. As this mom left the visit, the social worker explained how she would follow-up in 1–2 weeks to help set up the WIC visit once the application was processed. Some providers (and clinics) may wish to be even more ambitious, developing clinic-based food pantries so that next time Sandra comes to the clinic, she can receive a box of groceries to take home. These are all examples of how a provider might help a family in the office (Tier 1). Other, broader approaches illustrated below may complement this in-clinic action.

Tier 2. Community-Engaged Approach

For many families, public benefit programs may not be enough to fully support their needs. In our case, the father, Mateo, does not earn enough money each month to support his family's needs. Moreover, the family only receives a proportional amount of public benefits on account of Mateo's ineligibility. To make up this gap, providers have an opportunity to partner with key agencies and organizations. Such partnerships can support increases in parents' knowledge of available programs and reductions in barriers to access. Given the family's worries about Mateo's immigration status and their thoughts of disenrollment from SNAP and WIC, it is even more imperative that they are aware of community-based programs such as school meals, summer meals, local food panties, and hot meal sites that may exist across the community. In addition to developing strong partnerships with community agencies and organizations, providers can also be instrumental in engaging in larger community-wide efforts so that more schools, libraries, or other settings provide supplemental nutrition to at-risk families. Such activities, however, may need to be complemented with advocacy in support of FI-oriented policies and programs.

Tier 3. Advocacy-Based Approach

As noted in the case, Sandra and Mateo face numerous challenges on account of limited economic resources. We know that households that struggle with FI often face competing demands or priorities. For example, Sandra and Mateo likely struggle with the decision of whether to spend money on food or medical care for their children. The lack of consistent access to food and the parental stress that arises from having unmet food needs have significant negative effects on children's physical and mental health. Advocacy to address the families' FI will likely require more than providing services at the clinic visit and connection to community resources. It will likely require a broader perspective to address the root causes of the problems families face. For the provider seeing Sandra and her family in the clinic, advocating to address FI could take several forms. One method could be informing the local community of the struggles that families like Sandra face and advocating that local officials increase the resources available in the community. This could be to encourage the local government to increase the funding for food pantries in the area or improving families' access to local WIC offices. It could also come in the form of writing letters, as an individual or as a practice, to state and federal officials requesting increased SNAP and WIC benefits for families (Table 3.4).

Conclusions

This chapter examined the different types of responses that can occur when a patient or family is food insecure. We have shown how individual providers can respond to a positive FI screen in their clinical setting by giving information and linking families to resources. Providers can also collaborate with the larger community to address FI in a broader way while simultaneously advocating for key programs and policies that food insecure families rely upon.

References

1. Garg A, Dworkin PH. Surveillance and screening for social determinants of health: the medical home and beyond. JAMA Pediatr. 2016;170(3):189–90.
2. Chung EK, Siegel BS, Garg A, Conroy K, Gross RS, Long DA, et al. Screening for social determinants of health among children and families living in poverty: a guide for clinicians. Curr Probl Pediatr Adolesc Health Care. 2016;46(5):135–53.
3. Haggerty RJ. Abraham Jacobi, MD, respectable rebel. Pediatrics. 1997;99(3):462–6.
4. Perrin EC. Ethical questions about screening. J Dev Behav Pediatr: JDBP. 1998;19(5):350–2.
5. Garg A, Butz AM, Dworkin PH, Lewis RA, Serwint JR. Screening for basic social needs at a medical home for low-income children. Clin Pediatr. 2009;48(1):32–6.
6. Gottlieb LM, Hessler D, Long D, Laves E, Burns AR, Amaya A, et al. Effects of social needs screening and in-person service navigation on child health: a randomized clinical trial. JAMA Pediatr. 2016;170(11):e162521.
7. Kumar S, Preetha G. Health promotion: an effective tool for global health. Indian J Community Med. 2012;37(1):5–12.
8. Gold R, Cottrell E, Bunce A, Middendorf M, Hollombe C, Cowburn S, et al. Developing electronic health record (EHR) strategies related to health center Patients' social determinants of health. J Am Board Fam Med. 2017;30(4):428–47.
9. Ashbrook AH-GH, Dolins, J., Davis, J., Watson, C. Addressing food insecurity: a toolkit for pediatricians. Food Research and Action Center, American Academy of Pediatrics; 2017 Feb 2017.
10. Gottlieb LM, Tirozzi KJ, Manchanda R, Burns AR, Sandel MT. Moving electronic medical records upstream: incorporating social determinants of health. Am J Prev Med. 2015;48(2):215–8.
11. Thornton RL, Glover CM, Cene CW, Glik DC, Henderson JA, Williams DR. Evaluating strategies for reducing health disparities by addressing the social determinants of health. Health Aff (Millwood). 2016;35(8):1416–23.
12. Goddu AP, Roberson TS, Raffel KE, Chin MH, Peek ME. Food Rx: a community-university partnership to prescribe healthy eating on the south side of Chicago. J Prev Interv Community. 2015;43(2):148–62.
13. Bryce R, Guajardo C, Ilarraza D, Milgrom N, Pike D, Savoie K, et al. Participation in a farmers' market fruit and vegetable prescription program at a federally qualified health center improves hemoglobin A1C in low income uncontrolled diabetics. Prev Med Rep. 2017;7:176–9.
14. Savoie-Roskos M, Durward C, Jeweks M, LeBlanc H. Reducing food insecurity and improving fruit and vegetable intake among Farmers' market incentive program participants. J Nutr Educ Behav. 2016;48(1):70–6. e1.
15. Cohen AJ, Richardson CR, Heisler M, Sen A, Murphy EC, Hesterman OB, et al. Increasing use of a healthy food incentive: a waiting room intervention among low-income patients. Am J Prev Med. 2017;52(2):154–62.

16. Bowling AB, Moretti M, Ringelheim K, Tran A, Davison K. Healthy foods, healthy families: combining incentives and exposure interventions at urban farmers' markets to improve nutrition among recipients of US federal food assistance. Health Promot Perspect. 2016;6(1):10–6.

17. Buyuktuncer Z, Kearney M, Ryan CL, Thurston M, Ellahi B. Fruit and vegetables on prescription: a brief intervention in primary care. J Hum Nutr Diet. 2014;27(Suppl 2):186–93.

18. Carlson S, Rosenbaum, D., Keith-Jennings, B., Nchako, C.Center for Budget and Policy Priorities. Published September 29th, 2016. https://www.cbpp.org/sites/default/files/atoms/files/9-29-16fa.pdf.

19. Find Your Local Food Bank 2017 [cited 2017 November 13]. Available from: http://www.feedingamerica.org/find-your-local-foodbank/?_ga=2.102391489.1397199883.1504795425-1059098988.1488494947.

20. Greater Philadelphia Coalition Against Hunger website. Accessed December 2017. https://www.hungercoalition.org/.

21. Philabundance website. Accessed December 2017. https://www.philabundance.org/.

22. SHARE Food Program website. Accessed December 2017. https://sharefoodprogram.org/.

23. The Children's Advocacy Project. Accessed December 2017. http://cap4kids.org/.

24. Kaushal N, Waldfogel J, Wight V. Food insecurity and SNAP participation in Mexican immigrant families: the impact of the outreach initiative. B E J Econom Anal Policy. 2014;14(1):203–40.

25. Levedahl JW. How much can informational outreach programs increase food stamp program participation? Am J Agric Econ. 1995;77:343–52.

26. Schanzenbach DW. Experimental estimates of the barriers to food stamp enrollment 2009 November 13, 2017 [cited 2017 November 11]. Available from: https://www.irp.wisc.edu/publications/dps/pdfs/dp136709.pdf.

27. Bartlett S, Burstein N, Hamiliton W, Kling R, Andrews M. Food Stamp Program Access Study: Final Report. Food Assistance & Nutrition Research Program electronic publication. published November 2004. https://www.ers.usda.gov/publications/pub-details/?pubid=43407.

28. Crosnoe R, Fuligni AJ. Children from immigrant families: introduction to the special section. Child Dev. 2012;83(5):1471–6.

29. Jones MK, Bloch G, Pinto AD. A novel income security intervention to address poverty in a primary care setting: a retrospective chart review. BMJ Open. 2017;7(8):e014270.

30. Cosgrove S, Moore-Monroy M, Jenkins C, Castillo SR, Williams C, Parris E, et al. Community health workers as an integral strategy in the REACH U.S. program to eliminate health inequities. Health Promot Pract. 2014;15(6):795–802.

31. Murphy JS, Lawton EM, Sandel M. Legal care as part of health care: the benefits of medical-legal partnership. Pediatr Clin N Am. 2015;62(5):1263–71.

32. Palfrey JS, Hametz P, Grason H, McCaskill QE, Scott G, Chi GW. Educating the next generation of pediatricians in urban health care: the Anne E. Dyson community pediatrics training initiative. Acad Med: J Assoc Am Med Coll. 2004;79(12):1184–91.

33. Jones L, Wells K. Strategies for academic and clinician engagement in community-participatory partnered research. JAMA. 2007;297(4):407–10.

34. Wallerstein N, Duran B. Community-based participatory research contributions to intervention research: the intersection of science and practice to improve health equity. Am J Public Health. 2010;100(Suppl 1):S40–6.

35. Shalowitz MU, Isacco A, Barquin N, Clark-Kauffman E, Delger P, Nelson D, et al. Community-based participatory research: a review of the literature with strategies for community engagement. J Dev Behav Pediatr: JDBP. 2009;30(4):350–61.

36. Kania J, Kramer, M. Collective impact. Stanford Social Innovation Review [Internet]. 2011. Available from: https://ssir.org/articles/entry/collective_impact.

37. Edmondson J, Hecht, B. Defining quality collective impact 2014. Available from: https://ssir.org/articles/entry/defining_quality_collective_impact.

38. Earnest MA, Wong SL, Federico SG. Perspective: physician advocacy: what is it and how do we do it? Acad Med: J Assoc Am Med Coll. 2010;85(1):63–7.

39. Medical professionalism in in the new millennium: a physician charter. Ann Intern Med. 2002;136(3):243–6.
40. Education 2017. Available from: http://www.acgme.org.
41. Council On Community P, Committee On N. Promoting food security for all children. Pediatrics. 2015;136(5):e1431–8.
42. Law M, Leung P, Veinot P, Miller D, Mylopoulos M. A qualitative study of the experiences and factors that led physicians to be lifelong health advocates. Acad Med: J Assoc Am Med Coll. 2016;91(10):1392–7.
43. Interactive HTHP. Doctors, dentists, and nurses most trusted professionals to give advice 2009 [661]. Available from: http://www.harrisinteractive.com/harris_poll/index.asp?PID
44. Advocacy & Policy: American Academy of Pediatrics; 2017. Available from: https://www.aap.org/en-us/advocacy-and-policy/Pages/Advocacy-and-Policy.aspx.
45. Campbell EG, Regan S, Gruen RL, Ferris TG, Rao SR, Cleary PD, et al. Professionalism in medicine: results of a national survey of physicians. Ann Intern Med. 2007;147(11):795–802.
46. Gruen RL, Campbell EG, Blumenthal D. Public roles of US physicians: community participation, political involvement, and collective advocacy. JAMA. 2006;296(20):2467–75.
47. Minkovitz CS, Grason H, Solomon BS, Kuo AA, O'Connor KG. Pediatricians' involvement in community child health from 2004 to 2010. Pediatrics. 2013;132(6):997–1005.
48. Real FJ, Beck AF, Spaulding JR, Sucharew H, Klein MD. Impact of a neighborhood-based curriculum on the helpfulness of pediatric Residents' anticipatory guidance to impoverished families. Matern Child Health J. 2016;20(11):2261–7.
49. Klein MD, Alcamo AM, Beck AF, O'Toole JK, McLinden D, Henize A, et al. Can a video curriculum on the social determinants of health affect residents' practice and families' perceptions of care? Acad Pediatr. 2014;14(2):159–66.
50. Klein MD, Kahn RS, Baker RC, Fink EE, Parrish DS, White DC. Training in social determinants of health in primary care: does it change resident behavior? Acad Pediatr. 2011;11(5):387–93.

Chapter 4
Building and Evaluating the Impact of Food Insecurity-Focused Clinical-Community Partnerships on Patients and Populations

Adrienne W. Henize, Melissa Klein, and Andrew F. Beck

Abbreviations

CCHMC	Cincinnati Children's Hospital Medical Center
Child HeLP	Cincinnati Child Health-Law Partnership
FSFB	Freestore Foodbank
KIND	Keeping Infants Nourished and Developing
LASGC	Legal Aid Society of Greater Cincinnati
MLP	Medical-Legal Partnership
PDSA	Plan-Do-Study-Act
QI	Quality Improvement
SDH	Social Determinants of Health
SMART aim	Aim that is specific, measurable, achievable, realistic, and time-bound for a defined population
SNAP	Supplemental Nutrition Assistance Program
USDA	United States Department of Agriculture
WIC	Special Supplemental Nutrition Program for Women, Infants, and Children

Aims
1. Define the relationship between food insecurity, other potentially-related social determinants of health, and the drive toward population health equity.
2. Discuss critical components necessary to build and sustain successful community partnerships to address food insecurity.
3. Introduce quality improvement methods as a means through which interventions can be developed, evaluated, and sustained.

A. W. Henize (✉) · M. Klein · A. F. Beck
Cincinnati Children's Hospital Medical Center and University of Cincinnati College of Medicine, Cincinnati, OH, USA
e-mail: adrienne.henize@cchmc.org

© The Author(s) 2018   69
H. B. Kersten et al. (eds.), *Identifying and Addressing Childhood Food Insecurity in Healthcare and Community Settings*, SpringerBriefs in Public Health, https://doi.org/10.1007/978-3-319-76048-3_4

A Common Case in Primary Care Pediatrics

You are preparing to see your next patient, a previously healthy 9-month-old infant who comes into the primary care center for a well-child visit. The mother has no concerns about growth, development, or recent illnesses. Still, as you scan the screening questions completed at intake, you notice that the mother responded "yes" to your clinic's food insecurity (FI) question assessing whether she "worried that her food will run out and she will not have money to buy more." You glance at the child's growth charts and see they are all normal: weight, length, and head circumference are all stably between the 40th and 50th percentiles. In the exam room, you find the mother holding the baby on her lap. Another school-aged child is also in the room; this 7-year-old brother is on summer break. You start the visit, and the mother confirms that she does not have any concerns; she just needs an updated daycare form for the baby.

You first discuss common pediatric anticipatory guidance topics. Prior to starting your physical exam, you decide to explore the response to the FI question reported as positive on the intake questionnaire. The mother shares that the baby is enrolled in the Special Supplemental Nutrition Program for Women, Infants, and Children (WIC), but the formula supply she receives often runs out at the end of the month. The family generally uses their "food stamps," from the Supplemental Nutrition Assistance Program (SNAP), to buy more formula. The mother notes she works as a temporary employee, but 2 months ago, her employer reduced her work hours by 4–6 h per week for business reasons. She let the public benefits agency know of this decrease in her income, but her SNAP benefit did not change. Her housing and daycare costs also remained the same, leaving her with less money available at the end of the month. Now that it is summer, her older son does not receive meals at school, so her food bills have also increased. She has never been in this situation before and is not sure how she will make ends meet.

You move toward your physical exam. Happily, the infant is well appearing without any focal findings. You order the necessary vaccines and health maintenance labs. Knowing you need to provide counseling about FI, you consider the issues at the root of this family's challenges. How can you help? What are your in-clinic resources? What available community resources could help this family? Expecting that plenty of other families share a similar experience, you wonder what you and your practice could do to affect the entire community and a broader population.

Food Insecurity as a Key Social Determinant of Health

Let us start by considering the context in which our 9-month-old patient and her family grow, live, work, and age. FI, and other such risks, are themselves key determinants of subsequent health and well-being, potentially relevant to the myriad short- and long-term outcomes described in Chap. 1. Here, we suggest that FI may, too, be a marker of, or at least related to, other social, economic, and environmental factors with similar links to adversity. The World Health Organization defines the *social determinants of health* (SDH) as "the conditions in which people are born, grow, work, live, and age, and the wider set of forces and systems shaping the conditions of daily life" [1]. Put another way, the SDH are those "nonmedical factors influencing health." Such factors can be "downstream," including health-related knowledge, attitudes, beliefs, and behaviors. They can also, frequently, be "upstream" and include risks related to social, environmental, and economic realities or conditions (like FI) felt by patients and their households [2].

FI is a key "condition" that shapes the daily life of a child, family or household. Evidence also suggests that a single risk, like FI, is rarely felt in isolation. Patients (and households) experiencing one such risk frequently experience other similarly harmful risks related to the SDH. The accumulation of multiple such risks (e.g., being strained by FI plus housing and/or energy insecurity) results in the experience of steadily increasing adverse, undesirable health outcomes [3]. In short, the more SDH-related risks, the worse the outcomes.

Armed with this evidence, clinicians and practices are investing more time and energy into identifying and responding to household and community risks, like FI, that are rooted in the SDH [4]. It is becoming clearer that managing FI (and other SDH-related risks) is key to delivering effective, patient- and household-centered care that will result in the best possible short- and long-term outcomes [5, 6]. In pediatrics, there has been steadily increasing pressure to redesign care practices to more intentionally shine a light on these risks, normalizing their assessment and identifying relevant interventions that can appropriately address them [7, 8]. Without this more proactive approach, it should be no surprise that patients who are burdened by suboptimal conditions will grow, live, and age in ways that adversely affect their health and widen gaps between them and their less at-risk peers.

Food Insecurity, the Social Determinants, and Health Inequities

It is well established that individuals who experience risks like FI will, in turn, experience those health outcomes that we in the healthcare system strive to prevent. It follows that, in both the short- and long-term, such risks will drive disparities and widen health equity gaps. The potential for the SDH to influence health and well-being may be particularly profound for children as they find themselves growing and developing amid poverty and other potentially harmful conditions [9].

The terms health disparities, inequalities, and inequities are frequently used interchangeably. Recent discussions, particularly related to the concept of equity, have focused specifically on whether the distribution of resources matches the distribution of needs [10]. The World Health Organization defines *equity* as "the absence of avoidable or remediable differences among groups of people, whether those groups are defined socially, economically, demographically, or geographically."

Their companion definition for _health inequities_ centers on those differences in health-related outcomes that result from a "failure to avoid or overcome inequalities that infringe on fairness and human rights norms" [11]. Recall the established links between FI and the range of health outcomes of pertinence to health and well-being outlined in Chap. 1. An equity mindset would suggest that if risks like FI were effectively addressed, health outcomes could be improved; that is, those undesirable health outcomes could, and perhaps should, be remediable. In other words, if all households had equitable access to food – that is, need matched with resource – FI would be diminished. Additionally, adverse health outcomes resulting from FI could conceivably dissipate and outcome distributions would equalize.

Figure 4.1 will allow us to more deeply consider equity and the concept of matching need with resource specifically related to FI [12]. Figure 4.1a depicts three panels of shoppers at different food outlets. Each shopper is there to purchase groceries needed for their household. The individual on the far left has easy access to the items on their grocery list. They can easily see, reach, and place them in their cart. Moreover, the supply at this particular grocery store is plentiful, full of nutritious, high quality options. This household is likely food secure, with appropriate access to and availability of healthy food options. The individual in the center panel is having a little more difficulty. They can still see what they need, but they have a harder time reaching the items. When they do reach them, they must place them in a hand-carried basket, instead of a cart, that is growing heavier. The supply is less plentiful, and less appetizing, than that within reach of the shopper on the far left. Finally, there is the individual on the far right. This individual cannot even stretch to see the same items that the others can easily access. The supply is very limited with shelves generally stocked with less healthy, less appetizing options – perhaps this is a corner store and not a grocery store. Thus, they are forced to choose from what is available, less nutritious, more highly processed items. They do not have a cart or a hand-basket. Instead, they carry groceries in their arms while wrangling their small children; maybe they do not have access to child care. The two families on the right may represent families with food insecurity or at risk of food insecurity as their food access and availability is more limited than the family on the left.

The time spent in the store is only part of the shopping experience, however. Let us turn to Fig. 4.1b to consider challenges that follow these shoppers home. The person on the left has their own car. They quickly get home, unload their groceries, and carry on with their day. The individual in the middle rides the bus, carrying their packages with them on the journey homeward. The individual on the far right, along with their children, walks home, carrying heavy packages each step along the way. They will continue to have food needs even after their visit to the store, clearly a situation where their need, and the needs of their household, have not been met by the available resource.

Let us continue by picturing this third shopper at their home later that evening. Perhaps they are putting their 9-month-old infant, your patient, to bed. The infant may receive a bottle with formula diluted to make it last [13]. The mother may limit her own food intake because she was unable to get enough food to last the week. She may give her portion to her son or, perhaps, to another relative. This family's FI

a)

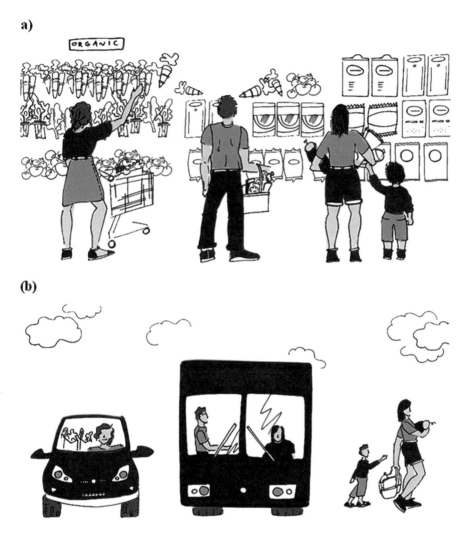

(b)

Fig. 4.1 Two visual depictions of the concept of equity in the context of (**a**) grocery shopping (availability of food); and (**b**) transportation to and from a food source (accessibility of food). (Credit: Alex Lohmann, BS (http://www.alexlohmanndesign.com))

could, therefore, be thought to result from "avoidable or remediable differences," factors that perpetuate the experienced risk while also influencing outcomes. It is, therefore, no surprise that certain individuals bear a disproportionate burden of adverse health outcomes. It is, similarly, no surprise that such individuals aggregate into populations that are far more challenged than others. As such, it naturally follows that issues of equity, and companion issues of social justice, can be considered at both the individual and population levels.

Food Insecurity and Population Health

Population health has been defined as "the health outcomes of a group of individuals, including the distribution of outcomes within that group" [14]. Embedded within this definition is a measure of both a health outcome and how that outcome varies within a defined population. Recall, once again, the 9-month-old infant introduced at the beginning of the chapter. Now consider this infant in the middle of a room filled with other infants her age. There will, naturally, be some variability with respect to how these infants are meeting their developmental milestones. Some may be crawling, some may be pulling themselves to a stand, and some may already be taking their first steps. Healthcare providers will naturally seek to maximize the potential for each one of these children, ideally having them all meet their milestones within the expected period of time. The concept of population health pushes us to similarly consider the underlying distribution. Although some variability is expected, this does not mean that some children are left behind. If the degree of variability, particularly that which is outside the bounds of what is considered normal, can be narrowed – by focusing attention on those in need while not neglecting the others – then actions should be taken. Indeed, the definition of population health has equity at its core, highlighting the importance of aggregate outcomes, but also ensuring that gaps in those outcomes are as narrow as possible [15]. It, therefore, demands a more effective match between need and resource.

Working toward this equitable need-resource match requires consideration of those factors influencing both outcome and outcome distribution [16]. Influential factors are frequently related to social determinants like FI and are at the root of what influences achievement of health equity [17, 18]. A focus on outcomes, and the equitable distribution of those outcomes, has pushed healthcare systems and communities in directions that may differ from traditional healthcare models. To start, the economic realities of health care have changed and are changing. With many providers (and practices) now existing within capitated, value-based payment models, there is growing pressure on achieving the best possible outcomes across patient panels [19–21]. This may require a shift in focus to adequately and effectively match need with resource, pushing risks related to the SDH to the forefront [22].

Mindful of this evolution, many professional organizations are pushing healthcare providers and systems in just this direction, encouraging actions that simultaneously address medical and social needs [8, 23]. The National Academy of Medicine highlighted this as a "vital direction," one that underscored the "central importance of social, behavioral, and environmental factors" across the life-course [24]. In line with this call for value and for equity, it follows that a prescription for food (or investment in FI reduction) may be just as important as a prescription for a medication. Changing incentives are changing the care landscape, and healthcare systems are focusing renewed attention on those determinants, social and medical, deemed to be of most pertinence to desired outcomes [25, 26]. This may be true even if those determinants, and their companion interventions, are well upstream of the outcomes in question [27].

If achieving population health equity requires upstream interventions targeting risks like FI, then innovative approaches to investment in the SDH will be required. Changing payment incentives may promote such investment but may also prove to be insufficient [28]. Indeed, there is currently a substantial imbalance in health and social service spending in the United States despite evidence suggesting that a re-balance could improve health outcomes [29, 30]. In lieu of short-term investment increases, it behooves providers (and practices) to consider how to best approach drivers of inequities in ways that improve outcomes and narrow gaps. Thus, a shift from thinking about the classical definition of a "medical home" to that of "health neighborhood" may facilitate development of novel strategies to address both individual and population health [31, 32].

Shift from Medical Home to Health Neighborhood for Individual and Population Health

Such a shift, from practice models that are medically-centered to family- or community centered, may benefit from a deeper understanding of the communities and populations served. In the realm of the SDH, it may benefit healthcare delivery systems, as key components of this "health neighborhood," to understand and partner with the community members and neighborhoods [33]. What are the social, economic, and environmental forces that affect individuals who walk through their doors? What are the realities faced on a day-to-day basis by the patients they serve? This shift requires a deeper understanding of risks and assets. Such factors may, themselves, influence how care can be more equitably delivered. They may also determine how providers can best design services in ways that effectively match need with resource [34].

An example of data that could inform care delivery is the place-based marker of a _food desert_. There are a variety of specific definitions and means of food desert identification, but there is still broad agreement about what the central concept represents. The United States Department of Agriculture (USDA) defines food deserts as "neighborhoods that lack healthy food sources." The USDA focuses on individual-level resources (e.g., income, vehicle accessibility), neighborhood-level resources (e.g., poverty rate, availability of public transportation), and accessibility to healthy food sources (defined by distance to a store or number of stores within an area) [35]. Specifically, the USDA defines low-income areas as those where the rate at which individuals live at less than the federal poverty level is at least 20%, the median family income is $\leq$80% of the state-wide average, or the median family income is $\leq$80% of the surrounding metropolitan area (if applicable). The USDA then defines areas as low access if at least 500 people (or at least 33% of the population) live more than ½ mile from the nearest supplier of healthy food if in an urban area or 10 miles in a rural area. Another classification uses a 1 mile distance in urban areas and 20 miles in rural areas [35].

Regardless of the specifics of how food deserts are defined, there is a tangible connection to the ability of individuals and households within a certain area to access what they need. Clinically, this has relevance because many may have difficulty acting on providers' advice to eat healthy food should they live in such a "desert." In other words, it may make perfect sense for a clinician to encourage their patients to eat more fruits and vegetables and less junk food; however, this may prove impossible if patients truly have limited access [36]. The photograph in Fig. 4.2 was taken in a neighborhood in close proximity to Cincinnati Children's Hospital Medical Center (CCHMC). This neighborhood is defined as a food desert given low income and low access, with no supermarket located within its boundaries. The photograph depicts the "produce section" in a local corner store, portraying a handful of rotten bananas and mostly empty shelves of poor quality fruits and vegetables. This lack of access is likely linked to the observed higher-than-average FI rates within the neighborhood. It is also likely related to higher-than-average rates of morbidity across a variety of conditions experienced by individuals within this neighborhood [37, 38]. With the goal of population health equity, medical homes and the broader healthcare system serving this neighborhood may benefit from the aforementioned shift to collaborative health neighborhood.

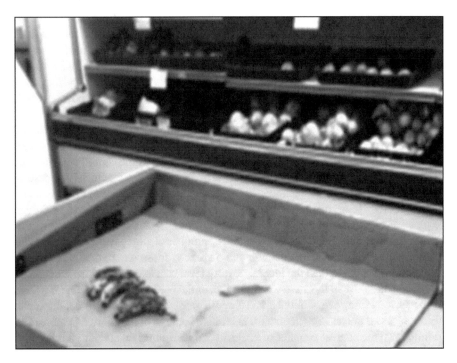

Fig. 4.2 A visual depiction of the "produce section" at a corner store in a neighborhood within Cincinnati, Ohio. (Credit: F. Joseph Real, MD MEd)

Such a shift requires a deeper understanding of equity across certain areas or populations. It also requires a deeper understanding of community assets, those partners that may be just as critical to improving health outcomes as any medically-centric intervention. Figure 4.3 depicts Greater Cincinnati's food deserts, those USDA-defined low income, low access census tracts or neighborhoods [39]. CCHMC, a large, academic pediatric medical center is depicted in the center of the figure. It is a tertiary care hospital as well as a primary care site for roughly 20,000 predominantly low-income children. This population of children experiences high rates of morbidity despite living in close proximity to the medical center. We posit that these outcomes stem, in large part, from the underlying conditions in which patients reside. As such, it should come as no surprise that there are several food deserts in close proximity to CCHMC. The circle surrounding the hospital, representing a 3-mile radius, captures a large number of such food deserts and is home to many of our patients. It also includes the corner store depicted in Fig. 4.2. But merely looking at this set of risks misses a key part of the story. Although there is plenty of risk spread across this region, there are also assets that are typically separate from the healthcare system. Within this depicted 3-mile circle are several food

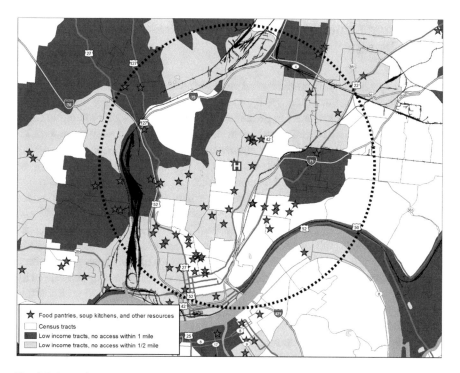

Fig. 4.3 Map of Cincinnati, Ohio depicting census tracts characterized as "food deserts." The map also depicts Cincinnati Children's Hospital Medical Center and a surrounding 3-mile radius illustrating those low income, no access tracts in close proximity, as well as food pantries, soup kitchens, and other resources. (Credit: Andrew F. Beck, MD MPH. Data sources: Freestore Foodbank, U.S. Department of Agriculture, U.S. Census Bureau)

pantries and soup kitchens that our patients may use. They represent key assets as well as potential partners in the drive toward achieving our collective goal of population health.

To achieve desired outcomes, there will need to be a variety of entities within this new concept of health neighborhood – hospitals and primary care clinics, as well as government, public, nonprofit, and private organizations across a range of sectors [40]. Moreover, it will require tighter linkages between healthcare systems (hospitals and clinics) and the communities they serve. This should prompt a deeper understanding of contextual factors, often rooted in the SDH, experienced each day by patients and patient panels [41, 42]. It should also prompt a shift from reactive management of disease to a more proactive, upstream approach to wellness and prevention. This has been called, by some, a "culture of health" that focuses on getting and staying healthy [43, 44]. Achievement of such a goal, particularly in an equitable fashion, will require short- and long-term management, or co-management, of both medical and social needs [45]. Indeed, medical treatment is unlikely to be successful should risks like FI compete for a patient's attention. This reality pushes us toward community collaboration and active community partnerships.

Prioritizing Clinical Interventions to Address the Social Determinants

While the current healthcare landscape calls for effective clinical-community linkages to optimize health outcomes for at-risk children, determining how and with which partners to collaborate can be daunting. Since children experiencing FI often simultaneously experience other risks detrimental to health and well-being, providers are challenged to prioritize interventions to address their patients' most pressing needs. Maslow's Hierarchy of Needs, familiar to providers in varied disciplines (Fig. 4.4), is one well-recognized framework that can help clinicians order risks and identify those community partners that share similar visions and strategies for addressing SDH [46, 47].

Maslow's Hierarchy highlights five levels of human needs considered essential to achieving one's full potential. These levels include food, shelter, safety, self-esteem and respect [46]. Families confronting issues like FI, denoted at the base of the Hierarchy, will often find it difficult to tackle issues farther up the hierarchy related to parenting or employment until that most pressing need is met. Recalling Chap. 2's lessons, it behooves clinicians to screen for multiple risks related to the SDH and then consider appropriate interventions to address families' self-prioritized needs. The most effective solutions will often include partnerships with families and community organizations that share common goals for the health and well-being of at-risk populations.

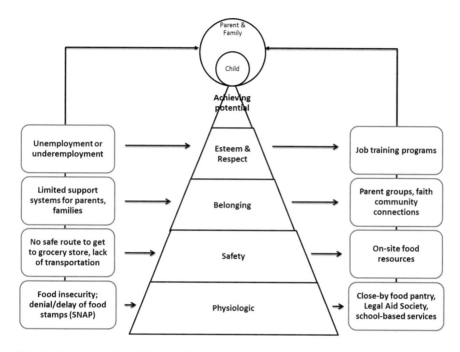

Fig. 4.4 Depiction of how Maslow's Hierarchy of Needs can be used to translate risks into connections to community resources. (Credit: Adrienne W. Henize, JD et al. [52])

Building and Sustaining Community-Based Interventions

Unlike medically-focused interventions that are still within the bailiwick of the healthcare system (e.g., referral from the primary care setting to a cardiologist), linking families to a community-based organization for an intervention focused on the SDH calls for more intentional strategies, processes, and commitment from both sides. Successful clinical-community partnerships require alignment around goals, leadership and resources, effective communication, processes that facilitate meaningful data sharing, and a plan to sustain and grow the collaboration [48–50]. Keeping this in mind, Fig. 4.5 illustrates an adaptable phased approach to building high-functioning partnerships between healthcare systems and the community. Such an approach can be highly complementary to the discussion of community-based interventions detailed in Chap. 3.

The first step, Phase 1, is to define the problem you are trying to solve [49, 51]. Logically, as a partner, you would seek out community hunger experts that share the clinic's vision of having healthier babies, children, and households who are not worrying about their food supply. This initial phase also includes consideration of what resources may be available to support a partnership. What will it take to move forward together? Are there funders who would support a joint application for a pilot

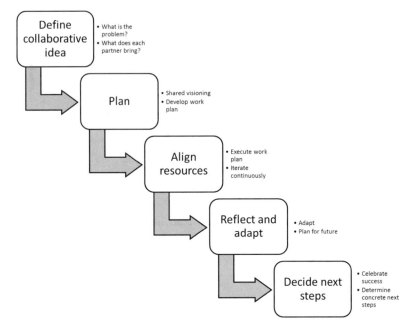

Fig. 4.5 A phased approach to community partnership development. (Credit: Adrienne W. Henize, JD et al. [52])

project? Do the healthcare and community organizations share any donors or board leadership who could help facilitate introductions and discussion?

Next, Phase 2 involves the development of an action plan with agreed-upon goals. What are you trying to accomplish together that you cannot do separately? As a healthcare organization seeing high rates of FI among its pediatric patient population, you might partner with a regional foodbank interested in addressing child hunger. The hospital has unique access to infants and children; the foodbank has the ability to provide formula to needy families. It is also essential at this stage to think strategically about what outcomes you could track to adequately assess progress towards your goals.

Resource alignment and implementation occurs in Phase 3. Here, you can see what works and what would benefit from refinement. Are there changes either partner can make to ensure families are being supported most effectively? In Phase 4, thoughtful reflection and adaptation can help ensure sustainability. For example, what data are you able to access and use together to further refine service delivery? Considerations in this phase might include whether funders are on board, if the intervention is effectively embedded in your practice, and whether you are training providers adequately to ensure the intervention is implemented routinely and effectively.

Finally, in Phase 5, continued growth and longevity of the partnership requires ongoing assessment and future strategic planning collectively by both partners. Can you spread to other clinics or populations? Also key is to acknowledge successes along the way. Sharing good stories with partners, media and with the broader community can help engender goodwill with stakeholders, including hospital leadership, donors, and families [52].

An Example of a Phased Approach to Building a Clinical-Community Partnership

The Cincinnati Child Health-Law Partnership (Child HeLP) is an example of how using this phased approach [52] can result in a successful, sustainable clinical-community partnership. Child HeLP is a medical-legal partnership (MLP) between CCHMC's primary care centers and the Legal Aid Society of Greater Cincinnati (LASGC). The partnership seeks to resolve civil legal issues common among low-income families (e.g., denial of public benefits such as SNAP, substandard housing, intimate partner violence) [53, 54]. Attorneys with expertise in poverty law are natural allies for clinicians caring for at-risk patient families with multiple such legal needs [55]. Early on, CCHMC and LASGC realized the two organizations shared a vision of child and family well-being and served very similar populations (Phases 1 and 2). Staff from both organizations then designed an intervention to most effectively serve families, including piloting social risk screening and referral procedures from the clinics to LASGC, strategizing about fundraising, and using quality improvement (QI) methods to track successes and implement changes (Phases 3 and 4). As this partnership nears its 10th year, CCHMC and LASGC continue to assess referral effectiveness, organizational capacity, and opportunities to expand (Phase 5). Using this phased approach, Child HeLP's referrals have steadily grown to >800 annually, with many positive legal outcomes for families [56, 57]. Next steps include piloting the MLP model in other vulnerable populations or settings. For example, Child HeLP is now facilitating the implementation of risk screening and legal advocacy within a hospital-based obstetrical practice to address legal issues affecting the health and well-being of pregnant women and their infants.

Of course, this framework can, and must, be adapted to fit the context within varied clinics and communities in order to be successful [58]. Regardless of the healthcare setting, clinicians can begin by assessing risk as explained in Chap. 2, identifying appropriate community partners like those identified here and in Chap. 3, and reaching out to organizations that share a vision for healthy children and families [50]. It is also essential to recognize the challenges inherent in partnership building, focusing on reaching solutions together. For example, lack of funding, reluctance of families or providers to engage in this kind of broader focus on SDH during clinical care, ineffective referral feedback, and lack of cohesive integration of the intervention into daily operations can derail even the most well-intentioned partnership. Trust, commitment and ongoing, meaningful conversation between partners can go a long way toward preventing such roadblocks while simultaneously supporting an intervention that can greatly affect at-risk families.

Using Quality Improvement Methods in Partnership Development and Assessment

Building and sustaining community partnerships could benefit from evaluation utilizing QI methods. Such partnerships exist at the core of the _Triple Aim_, which seeks to improve the experience of care for individuals, improve the health of populations, and reduce the per capita costs for all [59]. These bold objectives mandate innovation, identifying new and different ways to care for identified populations. The advent of QI methods in health care has provided a vehicle through which such innovation can be deployed and evaluated. Although a full review of QI methods is beyond the scope of this chapter, we will introduce certain QI concepts that are critical to moving toward achievement of a stated goal.

QI methods have their basis in the _Model for Improvement_. This framework guides on-going efforts by encouraging project participants to ask three critical questions: (1) What are we trying to accomplish? (2) How will we know that a change is an improvement? (3) What change can we make that will result in improvement? [60] These questions are central to the development of a specifically-targeted aim as well as the theory that serves as the basis for small-scale tests of change.

The first of the three questions serves as a valuable starting point – what are we trying to accomplish? What are we setting out to improve? This prompts the team to explicitly state their objective, often in the form of a _SMART aim_. Here, SMART is an acronym to guide aim development, encouraging the team to develop an objective that is specific, measurable, achievable, realistic, and time-bound for a defined population [60]. An example SMART aim could be, "to increase identification of household FI by the second-year pediatric residents working in the CCHMC Pediatric Primary Care Center from 1.9% to 15.0% within 6 months of project initiation" [61]. This was a SMART aim pursued at CCHMC at the start of FI-related in-clinic efforts.

Once such an aim has been defined, it is prudent to define measures critical to answering question #2 – how will we know that a change is an improvement? Generally speaking, there are three types of measures inherent to QI and relevant to this question. First, there is the outcome measure, that which is affecting the population of interest and which we are trying to change. Second, there are process measures, those steps along the way that are critical should the desired outcome be achieved. Finally, there are balancing measures which will help to identify whether any system changes result in new problems potentially popping up elsewhere [60]. Providing explicit operational definitions for each measure is vital for tracking progress.

Finally, we get to the third question – what change can we make that will result in improvement? Here, a frequent starting point is the development of a key driver diagram, a conceptual map that connects our aim to potential tests of change. These are connected by those key drivers, or essential factors, that are deemed likely to influence whether or not improvement is realized. Once this theory is established, it is time to start testing, often using the plan-do-study-act (PDSA) cycle model. PDSA cycles, targeting identified drivers, involve tests of change alongside consistent measurement to allow for an assessment of whether change results in improvement. First, team members plan out the test, identifying the objective, making predictions for what will happen, and determining how data will be collected during the test ("plan"). The test is then carried out during the "do" step. Measures highlight observations, positive and negative. These observations are analyzed during the "study" step, the learning phase to determine success and/or failures. These results then prompt action, leading to adoption of the tested change on a wider scale, adaptation for a subsequent test, or abandonment if the test was deemed ineffective ("act") [60]. Measurement is critical along the way, generally involving consistent tracking of outcome, process, and balancing measures over time. Run charts and statistical process control charts are often used to track such progress. Further information on these charts and QI methods in general is accessible and available through the Institute for Healthcare Improvement (http://www.ihi.org), a valuable resource for individuals and teams new to QI but committed to ongoing improvement [62].

An Example of Using Quality Improvement in the Clinical Setting

Keeping Infants Nourished and Developing (KIND), a clinical-community partnership created to address FI among households with infants seen in primary care, used QI methods early on to enhance identification of FI. Surveys of parents in CCHMC's primary care clinics confirmed an FI rate of 30% among households with infants younger than 1 year of age. The Freestore Foodbank (FSFB), the region's largest foodbank, had similar data reflecting high rates of FI among infants but lacked an effective means to address hunger in that population. CCHMC partnered with FSFB to address infant FI by distributing formula to families in need, training providers to screen for and identify FI, and supporting linkages for families to complementary community resources, including income stabilizing programs [6]. The partnership was built using the phased approach discussed earlier and QI methods described in more detail below.

When KIND was launched, pediatric residents at CCHMC were screening three out of four families for FI, but identifying less than 2% as food insecure. This prompted a QI project with the aforementioned SMART aim: to increase second-year pediatric residents' identification of FI from 1.9% to 15% within 6 months. In order to know if changes being tested resulted in improvement, the team defined their primary outcome measure as the percentage of households identified as FI by second-year residents during well child visits. The team then identified five key drivers thought likely to influence identification of FI households: (1) evidence-based criteria to standardize FI screening; (2) awareness about FI in the clinic population; (3) understanding of how and why screening is important; (4) residents empowered to intervene; and (5) buy-in from stakeholders.

Next came small tests of change targeting each driver. For example, to address the use of evidence-based criteria to systematically identify FI, a published 2-question screen was tested on paper, then embedded in the electronic health record (EHR) after early testing demonstrated its superiority to the existing screening tool. To drive awareness and understanding of FI among residents, several educational interventions were also tested, including a series of interactive multidisciplinary sessions focusing on the negative effects and prevalence of FI and the importance of effective screening. Run charts measured in time series were used to monitor improvement. During the six-month intervention period, residents' identification of FI increased from 1.9% to 11.2%, or from fewer than one family a week to almost five families a week [61].

This increase in FI identification was a key component of the initiation of the aforementioned KIND program. Now in its seventh year, KIND has distributed ~5000 cans of formula at the initial clinic site and spread to 12 additional sites across the region. Just as QI methods were used to enhance screening rates, so too have these methods been used to successfully implement and track this clinical-community partnership that now benefits thousands of families [6].

Conclusions

In this chapter, we defined key aspects of the social determinants of health, including food insecurity, and addressed concepts related to achievement of population health. In so doing, we highlighted the intersection between each of these critical topics and the movement toward equitable outcomes. We discussed how matching need with resource, risk with asset, often prompts the development of partnerships with key entities within the community. These partnerships, in turn, must be supported and grown in intentional ways, taking advantage of quality improvement methods to ensure they meet their objectives. Clinical-community partnerships are critical to meet the needs of patients and families and to help reduce the risks that can impair the health, growth, and development of patients like our 9-month-old and her 7-year-old brother introduced at the start of this chapter. Perhaps with an expanded view of our clinical responsibilities, with consistent and empathic screening, and with reliable and effective connections to community resources, we will more directly serve the needs of our patients and patient panels. Risks will be reduced and equity gaps will be narrowed for individuals and for populations.

References

1. Social determinants of health. 2017. http://www.who.int/social_determinants/en/. Accessed 25 May 2017.
2. Braveman P, Egerter S, Williams DR. The social determinants of health: coming of age. Annu Rev Public Health. 2011;32:381–98.

3. Frank DA, Casey PH, Black MM, Rose-Jacobs R, Chilton M, Cutts D, et al. Cumulative hardship and wellness of low-income, young children: multisite surveillance study. Pediatrics. 2010;125(5):e1115–23.
4. Hein K. Outside looking in, inside looking out–expanding the concept of health. Acad Pediatr. 2015;15(2):117–27.
5. O'Malley JA, Klett BM, Klein MD, Inman N, Beck AF. Revealing the prevalence and consequences of food insecurity in children with epilepsy. J Community Health. 2017;42(6):1213–9.
6. Beck AF, Henize AW, Kahn RS, Reiber KL, Young JJ, Klein MD. Forging a pediatric primary care-community partnership to support food-insecure families. Pediatrics. 2014;134(2):e564–71.
7. Coker TR, Moreno C, Shekelle PG, Schuster MA, Chung PJ. Well-child care clinical practice redesign for serving low-income children. Pediatrics. 2014;134(1):e229–39.
8. Council On Community Pediatrics. Poverty and child health in the United States. Pediatrics. 2016;137(4)
9. Blair C, Raver CC. Poverty, stress, and brain development: new directions for prevention and intervention. Acad Pediatr. 2016;16(3 Suppl):S30–6.
10. Braveman P. Health disparities and health equity: concepts and measurement. Annu Rev Public Health. 2006;27:167–94.
11. Health systems: equity. 2017. http://www.who.int/healthsystems/topics/equity/en/. Accessed 29 Jan 29 2017.
12. Kuttner P. The problem with that equity vs. equality graphic you're using. 2016. http://culturalorganizing.org/the-problem-with-that-equity-vs-equality-graphic/. Accessed 29 Apr 2017.
13. Burkhardt MC, Beck AF, Kahn RS, Klein MD. Are our babies hungry? Food insecurity among infants in urban clinics. Clin Pediatr (Phila). 2012;51(3):238–43.
14. Kindig D, Stoddart G. What is population health? Am J Public Health. 2003;93(3):380–3.
15. Marmot M, Friel S, Bell R, Houweling TA, Taylor S. Commission on social determinants of H. Closing the gap in a generation: health equity through action on the social determinants of health. Lancet. 2008;372(9650):1661–9.
16. Sharfstein JM. The strange journey of population health. Milbank Q. 2014;92(4):640–3.
17. Woolf SH, Braveman P. Where health disparities begin: the role of social and economic determinants–and why current policies may make matters worse. Health Aff (Millwood). 2011;30(10):1852–9.
18. Woolf SH. Progress in achieving health equity requires attention to root causes. Health Aff (Millwood). 2017;36(6):984–91.
19. Cheng TL, Emmanuel MA, Levy DJ, Jenkins RR. Child health disparities: what can a clinician do? Pediatrics. 2015;136(5):961–8.
20. Beck AF, Tschudy MM, Coker TR, Mistry KB, Cox JE, Gitterman BA, et al. Determinants of health and pediatric primary care practices. Pediatrics. 2016;137(3):e20153673.
21. Fierman AH, Beck AF, Chung EK, Tschudy MM, Coker TR, Mistry KB, et al. Redesigning health care practices to address childhood poverty. Acad Pediatr. 2016;16(3 Suppl):S136–46.
22. Woolf SH, Purnell JQ. The good life: working together to promote opportunity and improve population health and well-being. JAMA. 2016;315(16):1706–8.
23. Dreyer B, Chung PJ, Szilagyi P, Wong S. Child poverty in the United States today: introduction and executive summary. Acad Pediatr. 2016;16(3 Suppl):S1–5.
24. Dzau VJ, McClellan MB, McGinnis JM, Burke SP, Coye MJ, Diaz A, et al. Vital directions for health and health care: priorities from a National Academy of medicine initiative. JAMA. 2017;317(14):1461–70.
25. Baum FE, Begin M, Houweling TA, Taylor S. Changes not for the fainthearted: reorienting health care systems toward health equity through action on the social determinants of health. Am J Public Health. 2009;99(11):1967–74.
26. Wong WF, LaVeist TA, Sharfstein JM. Achieving health equity by design. JAMA. 2015;313(14):1417–8.
27. Williams DR, Costa MV, Odunlami AO, Mohammed SA. Moving upstream: how interventions that address the social determinants of health can improve health and reduce disparities. J Public Health Manag Pract. 2008;14(Suppl):S8–17.

28. Galloway I. Using pay-for-success to increase investment in the nonmedical determinants of health. Health Aff (Millwood). 2014;33(11):1897–904.
29. Bradley EH, Elkins BR, Herrin J, Elbel B. Health and social services expenditures: associations with health outcomes. BMJ Qual Saf. 2011;20(10):826–31.
30. Bradley EH, Canavan M, Rogan E, Talbert-Slagle K, Ndumele C, Taylor L, et al. Variation in health outcomes: the role of spending on social services, public health, and health care, 2000–09. Health Aff (Millwood). 2016;35(5):760–8.
31. Garg A, Sandel M, Dworkin PH, Kahn RS, Zuckerman B. From medical home to health neighborhood: transforming the medical home into a community-based health neighborhood. J Pediatr. 2012;160(4):535–6. e1.
32. Fisher ES. Building a medical neighborhood for the medical home. N Engl J Med. 2008;359(12):1202–5.
33. Kahn RS, Iyer SB, Kotagal UR. Development of a child health learning network to improve population health outcomes; presented in honor of Dr Robert Haggerty. Acad Pediatr. 2017;17(6):607–13.
34. Beck AF, Sandel MT, Ryan PH, Kahn RS. Mapping neighborhood health Geomarkers to clinical care decisions to promote equity in child health. Health Aff (Millwood). 2017;36(6):999–1005.
35. Food Access Research Atlas: United States Department of Agriculture; 2017. Available from: https://www.ers.usda.gov/data-products/food-access-research-atlas/documentation/.
36. DeMartini TL, Beck AF, Kahn RS, Klein MD. Food insecure families: description of access and barriers to food from one pediatric primary care center. J Community Health. 2013;38(6):1182–7.
37. Beck AF, Moncrief T, Huang B, Simmons JM, Sauers H, Chen C, et al. Inequalities in neighborhood child asthma admission rates and underlying community characteristics in one US county. J Pediatr. 2013;163(2):574–80.
38. Beck AF, Florin TA, Campanella S, Shah SS. Geographic variation in hospitalization for lower respiratory tract infections across one county. JAMA Pediatr. 2015;169(9):846–54.
39. Food Access Research Atlas. 2017. https://www.ers.usda.gov/data-products/food-access-research-atlas/documentation/. Accessed 4 Sept 2017.
40. Washington AE, Coye MJ, Boulware LE. Academic health systems' third curve: population health improvement. JAMA. 2016;315(5):459–60.
41. Purnell TS, Calhoun EA, Golden SH, Halladay JR, Krok-Schoen JL, Appelhans BM, et al. Achieving health equity: closing the gaps in health care disparities, interventions, and research. Health Aff (Millwood). 2016;35(8):1410–5.
42. Stine NW, Chokshi DA, Gourevitch MN. Improving population health in US cities. JAMA. 2013;309(5):449–50.
43. Hacker K, Walker DK. Achieving population health in accountable care organizations. Am J Public Health. 2013;103(7):1163–7.
44. Trujillo MD, Plough A. Building a culture of health: a new framework and measures for health and health care in America. Soc Sci Med. 2016;165:206–13.
45. Thornton RL, Glover CM, Cene CW, Glik DC, Henderson JA, Williams DR. Evaluating strategies for reducing health disparities by addressing the social determinants of health. Health Aff (Millwood). 2016;35(8):1416–23.
46. Maslow AH. A theory of human motivation. Psychol Rev. 1943;50:370–96.
47. Sameroff AJ, Seifer R, Barocas R, Zax M, Greenspan S. Intelligence quotient scores of 4-year-old children: social-environmental risk factors. Pediatrics. 1987;79(3):343–50.
48. Care P, Health P. Exploring integration to improve population health. Medicine Io, editor. Washington, DC: The National Academies Press; 2012.
49. Jolin M, Schmitz P, Seldon W. Community Collaboratives whitepaper: a promising approach to addressing America's biggest challenges. Washington, D.C.: Corporation for National & Community Service; 2012.
50. A Practical Playbook. Practical Playbook 2015. https://practicalplaybook.org/. Accessed 3 Feb 2015.

51. Toolbox Overview for Building Needle-Moving Community Collaborations. 2014. http://www.serve.gov/sites/default/files/ctools/CommunityCollaborativeToolkit_all%20_materials.pdf. Accessed 24 Sept 2014.
52. Henize AW, Beck AF, Klein MD, Adams M, Kahn RS. A road map to address the social determinants of health through community collaboration. Pediatrics. 2015;136(4):e993–1001.
53. National Center for Medical Legal Partnership. National Center for Medical Legal Partnership. http://medical-legalpartnership.org/. Accessed 23 Feb 2015.
54. Paul E, Fullerton DF, Cohen E, Lawton E, Ryan A, Sandel M. Medical-legal partnerships: addressing competency needs through lawyers. J Grad Med Ed. 2009;1(2):304–9.
55. Zuckerman B, Sandel M, Smith L, Lawton E. Why pediatricians need lawyers to keep children healthy. Pediatrics. 2004;114(1):224–8.
56. Klein MD, Beck AF, Henize AW, Parrish DS, Fink EE, Kahn RS. Doctors and lawyers collaborating to HeLP children--outcomes from a successful partnership between professions. J Health Care Poor Underserved. 2013;24(3):1063–73.
57. Beck AF, Klein MD, Schaffzin JK, Tallent V, Gillam M, Kahn RS. Identifying and treating a substandard housing cluster using a medical-legal partnership. Pediatrics. 2012;130(5):831–8.
58. Clinical-Community Relationships Evaluation Roadmap. Rockville, Maryland: agency for healthcare research and quality; Publication No. 13-M015-EF, July 2013. https://www.ahrq.gov/sites/default/files/publications/files/ccreroadmap.pdf. Accessed 29 Apr 2017.
59. Berwick DM, Nolan TW, Whittington J. The triple aim: care, health, and cost. Health Aff (Millwood). 2008;27(3):759–69.
60. Langley GJ. The improvement guide : a practical approach to enhancing organizational performance. 2nd ed. San Francisco: Jossey-Bass; 2009. xxi, 490 p.
61. Burkhardt MC, Beck AF, Conway PH, Kahn RS, Klein MD. Enhancing accurate identification of food insecurity using quality-improvement techniques. Pediatrics. 2012;129(2):e504–10.
62. How to Improve. 2017. http://www.ihi.org/resources/Pages/HowtoImprove/default.aspx. Accessed 31 July 2017.

Chapter 5
Developing an Action Plan to Fight Food Insecurity

Baraka D. Floyd, Deepak Palakshappa, and Melissa Klein

Abbreviations

AAP	American Academy of Pediatrics
CHILD HeLP	Cincinnati's Child Health-Law Partnership
EHR	Electronic Health Record
FI	Food Insecurity
KIND	Keeping Infants Nourished and Developing
MLP	Medical Legal Partnerships
QI	Quality Improvement
SDH	Social Determinants of Health
SNAP	Supplemental Nutrition Assistance Program
SWYC	The Survey of Well-Being of Young Children
USDA	United States Department of Agriculture
WIC	Special Supplemental Nutrition Program for Women, Infants, and Children

Aims

1. Outline the critical steps necessary to develop and implement a food insecurity program.
2. Discuss key partners and barriers to screening for and addressing food insecurity in healthcare settings.
3. Create an action plan to implement a program to reduce food insecurity.

B. D. Floyd (✉)
Stanford School of Medicine, Stanford, CA, USA
e-mail: bfloyd@stanford.edu

D. Palakshappa
Wake Forest School of Medicine, Winston-Salem, NC, USA

M. Klein
Cincinnati Children's Hospital Medical Center and University of Cincinnati College of Medicine, Cincinnati, OH, USA

© The Author(s) 2018
H. B. Kersten et al. (eds.), *Identifying and Addressing Childhood Food Insecurity in Healthcare and Community Settings*, SpringerBriefs in Public Health, https://doi.org/10.1007/978-3-319-76048-3_5

Introduction

As we consider moving forward to an action plan to fight food insecurity (FI), let us reconsider our case from Chap. 4. The provider treating this 9-month old, who lives in a food insecure family, can take steps to address this family's unmet food needs. The mere existence of such a family, though, leads us to recognize that this story may not be unique. With this recognition comes a call to action: developing, designing, implementing and evaluating a plan to fight FI at an institutional level.

Building the Case for FI Screening

One patient's or family's needs, assets, and barriers may make a compelling case to screen and address FI on an individual basis, but this may not be compelling enough to convince an institution or health care system to implement systematic FI screening. Since the family may or may not be similar to the population served at your institution, a needs assessment is often the first step to understand the issues faced by your patient population. A needs assessment can help identify the prevalence of FI among the patients seen at the institution and help understand the current institutional and community initiatives [1–4]. The needs assessment can take place at four levels, family, provider/health care team, institution, and community, and can create preliminary institutional buy-in.

Important Components of a Needs Assessment to Build the Case for FI Screening

The family or patient level needs assessment often begins in daily practice as providers notice patterns during day-to-day clinical care. A formal needs assessment can confirm what is seen in practice, provide a more complete understanding of the issue and resources to address it, and inform next steps [1, 2].While capturing the prevalence of FI in families at your institution is essential, determining what other social determinants of health (SDH), especially those at the base of Maslow's Hierarchy, are present in your population allows you to better identify the landscape of patient needs [1].Additionally, gathering information about structural barriers, (i.e. food deserts, poor public transportation) and individual level barriers (i.e. stigma and immigration fears) affecting families' access to food and resources is critical for developing screening practices and successful interventions [5–7].

Provider centered or clinic based needs assessments can also be beneficial in action plan development. Provider knowledge of and attitudes about FI burden at your institution can be examined for alignment with results from the patient and community needs assessment. Provider willingness to address FI is vital and should be included [1, 2, 7, 8]. In addition, key members of the health care team should be included in the initial provider or clinic based needs assessment.

The institution level needs assessment determines how any new action plan may fit into ongoing initiatives, institutional goals, and academic mission. What existing institutional efforts already exist to address FI or other SDH? Have other action plans been attempted, failed or discontinued, and if so, why [3]? Recognition of organizational values and strategic mission, such as value based care, innovation, or safety culture is an important consideration.

Patient, provider/health team, and institutional level needs assessments are complemented by ascertaining community organizations already addressing FI, since pediatricians will not be able to address FI alone. This model is similar to the model to care for a patient with complex medical issues where consulting a medical subspecialist to treat a condition correlates to consulting a community organization that addresses social complexity [1, 2, 8–10]. Since partnerships with community organizations are critical [2, 5, 8], recognizing the scope of local and regional community organizations that address FI is an important element of the needs assessment. Mirroring the ascertainment of other SDH, gathering information about programs and community organizations aimed at addressing these other SDH can influence innovative collaborations and provide a structure upon which to build an institutional action plan [1, 3, 11].While investigating what community organizations address the needs and barriers of your patients/families is critical to align resources with patient needs, it is also important to consider what organizations have capacity and desire to collaborate with the healthcare system.

Obtaining Preliminary Institutional Buy-In

An essential next step is convincing an institutional leader that addressing FI is important to gain institutional support and develop a strategy. Ideally, this is an exchange of information: you share the results of your needs assessment, and they advise on next steps in choosing key stakeholders and team members. This institutional leader can also assist with strategic alignment: how does addressing FI fit within institutional values or mission? Are there other ongoing initiatives onto which this plan could be mapped?

Choosing the proper leader at your institution is essential. This person should have decision-making power, accessibility, and understanding of the overarching institutional values, strategic mission, and initiatives. In *inpatient settings*, complex institutional structures and larger multidisciplinary teams are often difficult to navigate and engage. For this reason, administrative rather than clinical leadership may be best, especially if administrators carry more weight in making decisions. In *outpatient settings*, administrative or clinical leadership may share decision making power, so accessibility may be a key deciding factor in choosing a leader. Persuading this leadership figure requires that you share the results of your multi-faceted needs assessment and consider how FI fits into the organizational framework and mission. Vital to framing are linking FI to clinical outcomes addressed in that clinical area and demonstrating the potential to result in concrete benefits to families and the institution [3].

This institutional leader, your first key stakeholder, can help identify and enlist other key stakeholders. Traditional stakeholders include families [2, 12] medical providers (i.e. physicians, nurse practitioners), other licensed providers (i.e. dieticians, social workers, nurses), ancillary staff (i.e. community health workers, medical assistants), and community partners.

Development of a Collaborative Idea

Since providers and institutions will need to reach outside their walls to address FI, most ideas for action plans and programs are collaborative. To determine how and with whom to collaborate, one must first understand the strengths and weaknesses of their institution. This informs selection of key stakeholders and team members to implement your FI action plan. Table 5.1 considers four general types of institutions and the strengths and weaknesses that may exist.

Each institution has particular strengths that should be considered. Some are well established, while others may be discovered through your needs assessment and alignment with leadership. For example, if FI screening is already performed or resources are available in specific areas of the institution, these can be utilized to initiate your action plan. Additionally, prior institutional experience with implementing and sustaining interventions for SDH, such as medical legal partnerships (MLP) [15] or Health Leads [16], can provide a road map to building an action plan [3, 8].Given the need for collaboration in creating a FI action plan [1, 8], the presence of or willingness to build strong multidisciplinary teams and provider willingness to screen [2, 7, 8] are essential building blocks. Infrastructure such as a MLP to address immigration fears is helpful, since this is a known barrier to families accessing FI supports [5, 7]. Additional key elements of an action plan include provider training [7, 17], and system-wide quality improvement (QI) infrastructure [1].

In addition to strengths, challenges in a clinical setting must be considered while developing the action plan. Smaller settings may lack the personnel with diversity of expertise to compose a multidisciplinary team. Lack of knowledge about local resources, limited funding, and uncertainty about reimbursement may present as challenges to building and supporting the team [2, 7].

Identifying Your Team: On-Site Champion, Administrative Champion, Hunger Champion, and Community Partner

Prior to design and implementation of a robust collaborative idea, key stakeholders' views must be considered and strong team leaders identified. Integral team members, broadly defined, would include an on-site clinical champion, administrative champion, hunger champion, and a community partner.

Table 5.1 Strengths and weaknesses of specific clinical settings

Type of clinical setting	Academic institution	Large, multispecialty group practice	Community-based single specialty practice	Federally qualified health center
Strengths	• Multidisciplinary teams • QI infrastructure • Availability of internal funding streams • Medical-Legal partnerships • Access to other sectors promoting innovation: business, agriculture, design [13] • Access to patients • Access to community collaboratives and partners	• Availability of internal funding streams • QI infrastructure • Access to traditional model of multidisciplinary teams • More initiatives to draw from	• Familiarity and access to community collaboratives and partners • Fewer competing priorities	• Experienced in addressing SDH in high need population • Medical-legal partnerships • Access/participation in community collaborative
Weaknesses	• Productivity • Regulatory hurdles • Larger teams, more complex processes • Complexity of involving trainees • Various competing priorities: resident training, provider priorities [14] • Competing missions: high impact clinical work and scholarly productivity	• Funding • Productivity • Competing priorities of each individuals' "style" of practice	• Funding • Productivity • Lack of members for multi-disciplinary teams	• Funding: Compensating members of multidisciplinary team • Productivity • May lack resources to embed a program

The <u>on-site clinical champion</u> obtains buy-in from other participants and stakeholders in the practice or clinical setting with a commitment to address FI and ability to motivate and support their colleagues [3, 8].Their role also includes planning the essential steps of provider training [7], consistent communication and data collection. Ideally, they understand clinical flow and demands and can monitor how implementation affects these components. The on-site champion could be a physician, nurse, social worker, dietician or medical assistant. The <u>administrative champion</u>, possibly a clinic manager/coordinator or nursing supervisor, assures that the necessary supports for implementation are in place, such as physical space, electronic health record (EHR) support, and time and resources for training. In selection of a community partner, the community organization should share the same goal(s) as your clinical setting, and the strengths and weaknesses of the organization should complement those of your clinical setting. A <u>hunger champion</u> assures that the institution is up to date on policy changes, service availability, resources, screening tools, and other external aspects affecting the action plan in a specific clinical setting. The hunger champion can serve as a front-line contact for the community partner, and may be a volunteer, ancillary staff member, or another champion on the team, if they are able to fulfill to this role. Other team members can be selected based on your unique setting, with attention to those who can augment strengths and circumvent weaknesses.

Defining the Core Problem to Develop an Idea

Once the team is formed, the next step is to define the core problem and design potential interventions to address the core problem. Since our problem is FI, we would then use results from the needs assessment to further drill down the root causes of the problem. For example, if providers are uncomfortable asking about FI, it could be due to inadequate training, lack of an on-site social worker, or insufficient knowledge of community resources. In this case the core problem has three parts: lack of training to screen for FI, lack of in-clinic personnel to address uncovered issues, and inadequate knowledge of community resources. With a comprehensive definition of the problem, your team can define a shared mental model and vision. With your community partner at the table, you would galvanize around a goal [1, 2]. In this example, your team may decide that the goal is to increase provider comfort with screening and knowledge about FI resources. This allows the community partner to leverage their expertise and provide local resources to address FI. The administrative champion, on-site clinical champion, and hunger champion could disseminate this rich knowledge to medical providers and use it to guide implementation of FI screening in the clinical setting. Traditionally a social worker or community health worker have been added to address FI. However, incorporation of this ancillary staff may not be enough to lead to achievement of the goal of addressing FI. A robust collaborative team, with appropriate team members engaged in carrying out a plan that fully leverages one another's strengths with a shared mental model and goal is essential to success.

Plan

One evaluation framework to assist in developing and evaluating a new food insecurity program is the logic model. Logic models are visual tools that depict the relationships between an intervention's components and the intended outcomes [14]. A typical logic model consists of inputs, activities, outputs, and outcomes (Fig. 5.1). Inputs are the physical or financial inputs that go into a project. Activities are the actions of staff, providers, or community partners. Outputs are the direct result of the activities, similar to process measures. Outcomes are changes or results of activities and outputs. Logic models can convey the activities that make up an intervention, the relationships between those activities, and the link between the intervention and its intended outcome. Logic models have been widely used in public health and program evaluation since W.K. Kellogg Foundation published Logic Model Developmental Guide in 2001, and they are increasingly being used in quality improvement [18]. A clinical setting or practice interested in starting a food insecurity intervention could use a logic model to identify the critical components necessary to implement the program, how the program could fit in current practice workflow, and the process and outcome measures to identify in evaluating the program.

Key Components Necessary to Develop a Food Insecurity Program

While the specific components of a food insecurity intervention may depend on which activities are implemenedt based on the shared vision between the institution and their community partner, there are some components that every institution should consider/plan for at the outset.

A. **Screening**

Screening for FI is a key component of any plan and several questions emerge. First, consider *which FI **screening tool** works best for their site?* The American Academy of Pediatrics (AAP) recommends practices and clinical settings utilize the 2-item Hunger Vital Sign (Table 5.2) [9]. A response of 'often' or 'sometimes' to either question is considered a positive screen. Compared to the United States Department of Agriculture (USDA) 18-item Food Security Scale, this questionnaire has been found to have 97% sensitivity, 83% specificity, and is easier and more efficient to implement in a busy clinical setting. The Hunger Vital Sign has also been validated in both English and Spanish [9, 19].

Although the Hunger Vital Sign is recommended by the AAP, other questionnaires are available [2]. The Survey of Well-Being of Young Children (SWYC) includes one question ("In the past month, was there any day when you or anyone in your family went hungry because they did not have enough money for food") [20].

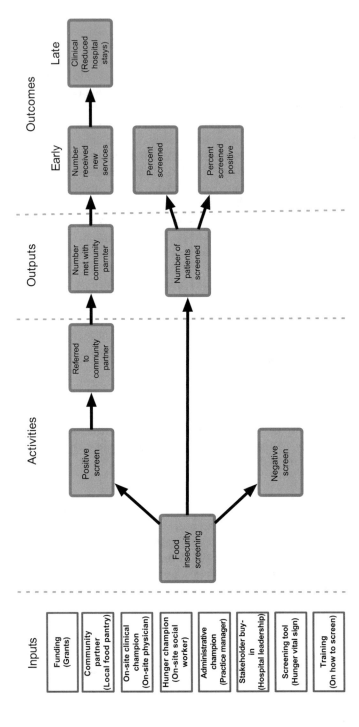

Fig. 5.1 Logic model for food insecurity related programs

Table 5.2 Hunger vital sign

Question	Potential responses
Within in the past 12 months, we worried whether our food would run out before we got money to buy more.	Often true, sometime true, never true
Within the past 12 months, the food we bought just didn't last and we didn't have money to get more	Often true, sometime true, never true

Second, **which patients and families** *should be screened for FI? Should a targeted or universal screening approach be implemented*? The AAP recommends that all patients be screened for FI at all routine health maintenance visits because FI and hunger often go unrecognized [9, 20]. Practices should consider their capacity and resources to address FI, but the literature favors universal screening, as demographic information, prior healthcare, and growth charts are poor predictors of food insecure households [21].

Third, **how** *will screening be implemented (electronically, paper-based, verbally)?* **Who** *will do the screening (physicians, nurses, ancillary staff)?* Practices will need to consider how screening will be best implemented into clinical workflow. This could be done verbally (a provider or staff member asks families presenting for a visit), written (a written questionnaire), or electronically (a tablet or kiosk in the waiting room). Prior studies have demonstrated that families prefer written or electronic screening; [22] however, practices will need to consider their clinic's workflow, families' literacy rates, and language preferences to determine the optimal system.

B. **Intervention**

A second key component that practices should plan for is the intervention. **What** *will the **intervention** include*? Each clinical setting will likely have different strengths and weaknesses (Table 5.1) to implement a sustainable model to address FI [2, 20, 23]. Although practices may not have capacity to dedicate sufficient staff time to connect all patients to the range of available nutrition or emergency food resources, there are multiple ways practices can promote and connect patients and their families to nutrition programs and food resources [24–29]. Table 5.3 lists some examples of activities that practices can do.

Utilizing the initial needs assessment, practices can determine what is most important for their patients/families and feasible for the clinical setting. Several key questions will emerge that need to be addressed early. **How** *will the clinical setting provide meaningful services for patients and their families*? The practice will need to decide whether they will provide services during the initial visit or point of care, or will someone follow-up (i.e. phone call, text, email) with the family after the visit. Providing services at the initial visit reduces the risk of loss to follow up and allows a warm handoff to community collaborators [11, 23, 29], but may be more time intensive. This also may not be feasible due to workflow constraints and or the ability of clinical setting to co-locate onsite services. **Who** *will provide resources for families*? Creating a sustainable model requires identifying and enlisting a <u>hunger</u>

Table 5.3 Food insecurity related activities in the clinical setting

Method	Example
Post information about federal nutrition program (Supplemental Nutrition Assistance Program (SNAP), Special Supplemental Nutrition Program for Women, Infants, and Children (WIC)) in your waiting room, exam rooms or bathrooms	Paper or electronic signs
Provide referrals to nutrition assistance programs or community partners	Provide families with a prescription for food or resources or a direct referral from your EHR
Provide application assistance in either initial application or denials or delays of benefits	Social work, community navigators, or benefits worker/food bank representative for initial applications Medical-legal partnership for denials and delays of benefits
Assign internal staff to assist food insecure families with accessing resources	Readily available websites and lists of pantries sorted by zip code/neighborhood
Integrate a community partner in the practice to provide point-of-care services	Health leads, benefit worker or food bank representative, community navigators

champion who can connect families to nutrition assistance programs (e.g. SNAP, WIC). This individual could be a clinical staff member (e.g. social worker, physician, nurse, medical assistant, community health worker), member of a community partner organization, or a long-term volunteer. The hunger champion's role should also include helping the clinical setting remain up to date on changes in nutrition policy changes and screening procedures to assist the practice in developing a sustainable FI intervention [20].

Execute Plan and Evaluate Progress

After the team decides on the intervention and creates an action plan, which includes a shared vision with short and long-term goals, the next step is to execute the plan. As part of their action plan, practices and clinical settings should include a means to consistently track data to ensure the goals are reached [1]. These metrics can be assessed formally through quality improvement initiatives or implementation science (see Chap. 4). Consistent evaluation using shared data is necessary to further the partnership's vision and goals, hopefully leading to improved health. Data tracking should include process measures (e.g. number of families screened or referred to a specific resource), outcome metrics (e.g. number of families who receive a SNAP) and population health metrics (i.e. FI rate across the community). Clearly, the process, patient and population level outcomes metrics assessed are dependent on the model implemented (e.g. physicians provide referrals, integrating a community partner in the practice); thus, a detailed plan or logic model that includes the critical steps of the program can help identify the important short and long-term steps to evaluate. Assessing these different levels of metrics is important to inform on the effectiveness of the FI program and ensure that the intervention is impacting those it is intended to help.

Potential Domains for Evaluation: Screening and Intervention Outcomes

The AAP has recommended that clinicians screen all patients presenting for routine health maintenance visits [9]. Assessment of screening rates is critical to ensure that patients are screened as planned. Incorporating screening in the EHR can serve as a prompt to remind clinicians to screen but also allows for more reliable tracking of the data. Once the clinical setting can determine that the patients are reliably screened, the next process measure is to determine the effectiveness of screening. Consistent screening without detection of FI may represent an issue in the screening process (i.e. inappropriate screen, need to screen in alternate format) or the need to provide additional training on empathic screening (see Chap. 2 for training). Whether screening is done electronically or verbally, providers should document results in the EHR. Documenting results in the patient's medical record can assist in future patient care, informing providers who will see the patient at subsequent visits. The Hunger Vital Sign is already built into the Epic Foundation System and can be used to assist in monitoring positive screens. With its new SDH platform comes the ability to document a SDH problem list, integrate resources and resource referrals, and see prior screening results through the same feature allowing medical records to be viewed between different EPIC systems [30]. The ICD-10-CM Diagnosis Code Z59.4 (lack of adequate food and safe drinking water) can also be used to document FI on the patient's problem list [20].

   Equally important as evaluation of screening rates is assessment of the interventions for identified families. Clearly, this will depend on the previously decided upon intervention strategy (e.g. provide a list of community resources, application for SNAP). Regardless of the intervention, assessment of consistency that the resources are provided and community connections made is critical. Documentation of screening and intervention provides a means to follow patients longitudinally (e.g. family was provided a list of local food pantries, mother met with community partner to discuss SNAP benefits). After assessing the resources and referrals provided during the index visit, the collaboration should evaluate whether the family accessed that resource and received the expected services. As the goal of these programs is to connect families to reduce FI, it is important to measure if families receive the expected support and outcomes from the resource and referral. Developing a process to track referrals to community resources and applications for federal nutrition programs will provide important information about the program's efficacy. During the planning phase of the intervention, patient privacy from both the medical (i.e. HIPAA) and community partner's perspective should be addressed. Routine and transparent sharing of meaningful data are critical to identifying opportunities and barriers to achieving the intended outcomes. Active data tracking can also provide an opportunity to address systemic issues that affect families that would otherwise go unrecognized (e.g. transportation, public policy changes) and plan next steps.

Utilizing Data to Drive Next Steps

Systematic tracking of processes, patient, family, and population health outcomes can be instrumental in determining next steps. Providers, practices, clinical settings, and community partners can use this data to assess the progress of the program, identify new opportunities affecting food insecure families, and advocate for new programs to address families' unmet needs.

Measuring and analyzing both process and outcome measures can directly be used to ensure that the intervention is reaching the intended families, identify barriers impeding desired outcomes and assess the program's impact on patients as well as the larger population. This deliberate focus on data and outcomes can lead to tailored interventions that better address the families' needs and efforts to advocate for larger systematic changes.

Case Example 1 *Evaluation of process and outcome measures shifts to intervention to better meet families' needs*

A study of six suburban pediatric primary care practices that implemented FI screening [22, 31] found that the planned interventions were not resulting in the expected outcomes. Families who screened positive were eligible to be referred to a community partner to assist them in applying for SNAP benefits. In the first 6 months of the screening program, 122 families screened positive for FI, but only one of those families received new SNAP benefits. Further programmatic evaluation revealed that over 75% of families who were eligible were screened by clinicians, but only 9 of the families who screened positive talked to the community partner. Qualitative work, with the clinicians and families, identified that many families who screened positive were either already receiving appropriate SNAP benefits or already reviewed eligibility criteria and knew they were not eligible. The practices used this data to modify the FI intervention to also provide families with information about local food resources (e.g. food pantries in the area).

Identifying New Opportunities

Continuously tracking measures and sharing data can also help partnerships identify new opportunities to assist families. As programs progress, there may be unanticipated systematic barriers or issues that arise. Once identified, practices and community partners can collaboratively address issues which may enhance the effectiveness of the program or lead to the development of new programs [1]. One example is Cincinnati's Child Health-Law Partnership (Child HeLP), the medical legal partnership between Cincinnati Children's Hospital primary care centers and the Legal Aid Society of Greater Cincinnati. Physicians and attorneys work together to identify families with public benefit denials and delays, one of the root causes of FI. Physicians recognized that many of their families with infants were food insecure despite appropriate SNAP and WIC and as a result, formula stretching practices were commonly used to make ends meet [32]. To meet these newly discovered needs, a new program was built with the FreeStore FoodBank, the area's largest food bank. The program, Keeping Infants Nourished and Developing (KIND), was established to allow the provision of formula to infants in FI families. With implementation of the KIND program, additional screening [24] to target infants was required and subsequent evaluation [8] of patient outcomes led to programmatic expansion.

Advocacy

In order to address child hunger, the AAP recommends that clinicians support advocacy to end child FI. Pediatricians have a long history of advocating for policies to improve child nutrition and the overall health at the local, state, or federal levels. As discussed in Chap. 3, there are multiple ways in which providers can advocate to end child FI (e.g. directly reaching out to policy makers, summarizing data for lay audiences). The data gathered from evaluating a clinical setting's program could also be used in advocacy efforts. For example, it could be useful to inform local community leaders about the prevalence of FI or lawmakers about the importance of supporting policies that address child hunger (e.g. SNAP, WIC).

Sustainability

To ensure the sustainability of the FI intervention, practices and their community partners need to consider the financial structure and programmatic funding. Establishing effective FI screening processes, embedding programs within practices, and coordinating care with community partners often requires reliable funding streams. With national organizations and payers increasingly moving to value-based payment models, rather than fee for service, visit based reimbursement structure may provide increasing opportunities to implement FI interventions in clinical practices [2]. As discussed in Chap. 2, the Centers for Medicare and Medicaid recently provided funding for Accountable Health Communities, which are designed to address the gap between clinical care and community services and represent increasing support for new models of care. This type of model may be adapted by other Accountable Care Organizations to provide funding for care coordination that would address FI as well as the other social determinants. Continuously tracking data on outcome measures that lead to improved health, potentially with decreased cost, could garner support from government or private payers to pursue additional innovative care models.

Summary

In this chapter, we discuss some the critical steps necessary to develop an effective and sustainable FI program. Creating an action plan that includes strengths and weaknesses of the institution is important. This action plan can then be utilized to identify key stakeholders and partners, determine the core problems and steps to address them, and incorporate an evaluation process from the outset. We believe that following the blueprint outlined will assist a clinical setting or institution interested in implementing a FI program.

References

1. Henize AW, Beck AF, Klein MD, Adams M, Kahn RS. A road map to address the social determinants of health through community collaboration. Pediatrics. 2015;136(4):e993–1001.
2. Fierman AH, Beck AF, Chung EK, Tschudy MM, Coker TR, Mistry KB, et al. Redesigning health care practices to address childhood poverty. Acad Pediatr. 2016;16(3):S136–46.
3. Zuckerman B. Growing up poor: a pediatric response. Acad Pediatr. 2014;2014(14):431–5.
4. Wright J, Williams R, Wilkinson JR. Development and importance of health needs assessment. BMJ. 1998;316(7140):1310–3.
5. Bruce JS, Cruz MMDL, Moreno G, Chamberlain LJ. Lunch at the library: examination of a community-based approach to addressing summer food insecurity. Public Health Nutr. 2017;20(9):1640–9.
6. Kaiser L. Why do low-income women not use food stamps? Findings from the California Women's health survey. Public Health Nutr. 2008;11(12):1288.
7. Barnidge E, LaBarge G, Krupsky K, Arthur J. Screening for food insecurity in pediatric clinical settings: opportunities and barriers. J Community Health. 2017;42(1):51–7.
8. Beck AF, Henize A, Kahn RS, Reiber KL, Young JJ, Klein MD. Forging a Pediatric Primary Care-Community Partnership to Support Food-Insecure Families. Pediatrics. 2014;134(2):e564–71.
9. Council on Community Pediatrics C on N. Promoting food security for all children. Pediatrics. 2015;136(5):e1431–8.
10. Community Pediatrics C on. Community pediatrics: navigating the intersection of medicine, public health, and social determinants of children's health. Pediatrics. 2013;131(3):623–8.
11. Sandel M, Hansen M, Kahn R, Lawton E, Paul E, Parker V, et al. Medical-legal partnerships: transforming primary care by addressing the legal needs of vulnerable populations. Health Aff (Millwood). 2010;29(9):1697–705.
12. Flacks J, Boynton-Jarret R. Strengths-based approaches to screening families for health-related social needs in the healthcare setting: preview of recommendations. 2017. https://www.cssp.org/publications/documents/Strengths-based-Screening-Preview-Recommendations.pdf. Accessed 3 Oct 2017.

13. Block DR, Thompson M, Euken J, Liquori T, Fear F, Baldwin S. Engagement for transformation: value webs for local food system development. Agric Hum Values. 2008;25(3):379–88.
14. Kenyon CC, Palakshappa D, Feudtner C. Logic models–tools to bridge the theory-research-practice divide. JAMA Pediatr. 2015;169(9):801–2.
15. National Center for Medical-Legal Partnership. National Center for Medical-Legal Partnership. http://medical-legalpartnership.org/. Accessed 17 Nov 2017.
16. Health Leads. Health leads. https://healthleadsusa.org/. Accessed 17 Nov 2017.
17. Beck AF, Henize A, Kahn RS, Reiber K, Klein MD. Curtailing food insecurity with clinical-community collaboration. 2015. http://healthaffairs.org/blog/2015/07/09/curtailing-food-inse-curity-with-clinical-community-collaboration/. Accessed 17 Sept 2017.
18. Siriwardena AN, Gillam S. Understanding processes and how to improve them. Qual Prim Care. 2013;21(3):179–85.
19. Hager ER, Quigg AM, Black MM, Coleman SM, Heeren T, Rose-Jacobs R, et al. Development and validity of a 2-item screen to identify families at risk for food insecurity. Pediatrics. 2010;126(1):e26–32.
20. Addressing food insecurity: a toolkit for pediatricians. Food Research & Action Center. http://frac.org/aaptoolkit. Accessed 27 Oct 2017.
21. Palakshappa D, Khan S, Feudtner C, Fiks AG. Acute health care utilization among food-insecure children in primary care practices. J Health Care Poor Underserved. 2016;27(3):1143–58.
22. Palakshappa D, Doupnik S, Vasan A, Khan S, Seifu L, Feudtner C, et al. Suburban families' experience with food insecurity screening in primary care practices. Pediatrics. 2017;140(1):e20170320.
23. Beck AF, Tschudy MM, Coker TR, Mistry KB, Cox JE, Gitterman BA, et al. Determinants of health and pediatric primary care practices. Pediatrics. 2016;137(3)
24. Burkhardt MC, Beck AF, Conway PH, Kahn RS, Klein MD. Enhancing accurate identification of food insecurity using quality-improvement techniques. Pediatrics. 2012;129(2):e504–10.
25. Fleegler EW, Lieu TA, Wise PH, Muret-Wagstaff S. Families' health-related social problems and missed referral opportunities. Pediatrics. 2007;119(6):e1332–41.
26. Garg A, Toy S, Tripodis Y, Silverstein M, Freeman E. Addressing social determinants of health at well child care visits: a cluster RCT. Pediatrics. 2015;135(2):e296–304.
27. DeMartini TL, Beck AF, Kahn RS, Klein MD. Food insecure families: description of access and barriers to food from one pediatric primary care center. J Community Health. 2013;38(6):1182–7.
28. Klein MD, Alcamo AM, Beck AF, O'Toole JK, McLinden D, Henize A, et al. Klein 2014. Can a video curriculum on the social determinants of health affect residents' practice and families' perceptions of care? Acad Pediatr. 2014;14(2):159–66.
29. Gottlieb LM, Hessler D, Long D, Laves E, Burns AR, Amaya A, et al. Effects of social needs screening and in-person service navigation on child health: a randomized clinical trial. JAMA Pediatr. 2016;170(11):e162521.
30. PRAPARE EPIC Training. http://www.nachc.org/wp-content/uploads/2016/07/PRAPARE-Epic-Training.pdf. Accessed 1 Dec 2017.
31. Palakshappa D, Vasan A, Khan S, Seifu L, Feudtner C, Fiks AG. Clinicians' perceptions of screening for food insecurity in suburban pediatric practice. Pediatrics. 2017;140(1)
32. Burkhardt MC, Beck AF, Kahn RS, Klein MD. Are our babies hungry? Food insecurity among infants in urban clinics. Clin Pediatr (Phila). 2012;51(3):238–43.

Index

© The Author(s) 2018
H. B. Kersten et al. (eds.), *Identifying and Addressing Childhood Food
Insecurity in Healthcare and Community Settings*, SpringerBriefs in Public
Health, https://doi.org/10.1007/978-3-319-76048-3

Printed in the United States
By Bookmasters